ETHICS, HEALTH ... ... PUBLIC

Public health is . ... of ethical discussion.
In this volume a rang... ... ethics are explored using
the resources of moral theory, ...cal philosophy, philosophy of science,
applied ethics, law, and economics.

The twelve original papers presented consider numerous ethical issues
arise within public health ethics. To what extent can the public good or
the public interest justify state interventions that impose limits upon the
freedom of individuals? What role should the law play in regulating risks?
Should governments actively aim to change our preferences about such
things as food, smoking or physical exercise? What are public goods, and what
role (if any) do they play in public health? To what extent do individuals
have moral obligations to contribute to protecting the community or the
public good? Where is it appropriate to concentrate upon prevention rather
than cure? Given the fact that we cannot be protected from all harm, what
sorts of harm provide a justification for public health action? What limits
do we wish to place upon public health activities? How do we ensure that
the interests of individuals are not set aside or forgotten in the pursuit of
population benefits?

An excellent line-up of authors from North America, Europe, and the
UK tackle these questions.

Angus Dawson is Senior Lecturer in Ethics at the Center for Professional
Ethics at Keele University

Marcel Verweij is Associate Professor at the Ethics Institute at Utrecht
University

ISSUES IN BIOMEDICAL ETHICS

General Editors
John Harris and Søren Holm

Consulting Editors
Raanan Gillon and Bonnie Steinbock

The late twentieth century witnessed dramatic technological developments in biomedical science and in the delivery of health care, and these developments have brought with them important social changes. All too often ethical analysis has lagged behind these changes. The purpose of this series is to provide lively, up-to-date, and authoritative studies for the increasingly large and diverse readership concerned with issues in biomedical ethics—not just health care trainees and professionals, but also philosophers, social scientists, lawyers, social workers, and legislators. The series will feature both single-author and multi-author books, short and accessible enough to be widely read, each of them focused on an issue of outstanding current importance and interest. Philosophers, doctors, and lawyers from a number of countries feature among the authors lined up for the series.

Ethics, Prevention, and Public Health

EDITED BY

Angus Dawson and Marcel Verweij

CLARENDON PRESS · OXFORD

OXFORD
UNIVERSITY PRESS

Great Clarendon Street, Oxford ox2 6DP

Oxford University Press is a department of the University of Oxford.
It furthers the University's objective of excellence in research, scholarship,
and education by publishing worldwide in

Oxford New York

Auckland Cape Town Dar es Salaam Hong Kong Karachi
Kuala Lumpur Madrid Melbourne Mexico City Nairobi
New Delhi Shanghai Taipei Toronto

With offices in

Argentina Austria Brazil Chile Czech Republic France Greece
Guatemala Hungary Italy Japan Poland Portugal Singapore
South Korea Switzerland Thailand Turkey Ukraine Vietnam

Oxford is a registered trade mark of Oxford University Press
in the UK and in certain other countries

Published in the United States
by Oxford University Press Inc., New York

British Library Cataloguing in Publication Data
Data available

Library of Congress Cataloging in Publication Data
Data available

Typeset by Laserwords Private Limited, Chennai, India
Printed in Great Britain
on acid-free paper by the
MPG Books Group, Bodmin and King's Lynn

ISBN 978–0–19–929069–7 (Hbk.)
ISBN 978–0–19–957053–9 (Pbk.)

10 9 8 7 6 5 4 3 2 1

CONTENTS

Notes on Contributors   vii

Preface   xi

1. Introduction: Ethics, Prevention, and Public Health   1
   Angus Dawson and Marcel Verweij

2. The Meaning of 'Public' in 'Public Health'   13
   Marcel Verweij and Angus Dawson

3. Public Health and Civic Republicanism: Toward an
   Alternative Framework for Public Health Ethics   30
   Bruce Jennings

4. Health of the People: The Highest Law?   59
   Lawrence O. Gostin and Lesley Stone

5. Population-Level Bioethics: Mapping a New Agenda   78
   Daniel Wikler and Dan W. Brock

6. Parental Choice and Expert Knowledge in the Debate about
   MMR and Autism   95
   Tom Sorell

7. Ethical Issues in Applying Quantitative Models for Setting
   Priorities in Prevention   111
   Dan W. Brock

8. Reasonable Limits to Public Health Demands   129
   Mariëtte van den Hoven

 9. Vertical Transmission of Infectious Diseases and Genetic
    Disorder: Are the Medical and Public Responses Consistent?   145
    **Jay A. Jacobson, Margaret P. Battin, Jeffrey R. Botkin,
    Leslie Francis, James O. Mason, and Charles B. Smith**

10. Herd Protection as a Public Good: Vaccination and our
    Obligations to Others   160
    Angus Dawson

11. Tobacco Discouragement: A Non-Paternalistic Argument   179
    Marcel Verweij

12. Informed Consent and the Expansion of Newborn Screening   198
    Niels Nijsingh

    References   213
    Index   233

NOTES ON CONTRIBUTORS

Margaret P. Battin, MFA, PhD, is Distinguished Professor in the Department of Philosophy at the University of Utah; and Adjunct Professor in the Division of Medical Ethics, Department of Internal Medicine at the University of Utah School of Medicine. Current areas of interest and research include suicide, physician-assisted suicide and euthanasia, ethics and infectious disease, and reproductive rights.

Jeffrey R. Botkin, MD, MPH, is Professor of Pediatrics in the Department of Pediatrics; Adjunct Professor of Medicine for the Division of Medical Ethics in the Department of Internal Medicine, University of Utah School of Medicine; and Associate Vice President for Research Integrity at the University of Utah. Current areas of interest and research include research ethics, newborn screening, genetic testing and prenatal diagnosis.

Dan W. Brock is the Frances Glessner Lee Professor of Medical Ethics in the Department of Social Medicine; Director of the Division of Medical Ethics at the Harvard Medical School; and Director of the Harvard University Program in Ethics and Health. He is the author of over 150 articles on various topics in bioethics, and moral and political philosophy. He is the author of *Deciding For Others: The Ethics of Surrogate Decision Making* (1989) (with Allen E. Buchanan), *Life and Death: Philosophical Essays in Biomedical Ethics*, (1993), and *From Chance to Choice: Genetics and Justice* (2000) (with Allen Buchanan, Norman Daniels and Daniel Wikler).

Angus Dawson is currently Senior Lecturer in Ethics and Philosophy in the Centre for Professional Ethics at Keele University in the UK. His main research interests are in public health ethics (particularly vaccinations) and the use of empirical evidence in moral arguments.

Leslie Francis, PhD, JD, is Professor of Philosophy and the Alfred C. Emery Professor of Law; Adjunct Professor of Political Science at the University of

Utah; and Adjunct Professor in the Division of Medical Ethics, Department of Internal Medicine at the University of Utah School of Medicine. Current areas of interest and research include bioethics and the law of bioethics, health law, the philosophy of law, and research ethics.

Lawrence O. Gostin is Professor of Law and Associate Dean at Georgetown University; Professor of Law and Public Health at The Johns Hopkins University; and Director at the Center for Law and the Public's Health (A WHO and CDC Collaborating Center). He is the author of numerous papers and books including the influential volume, *Public Health Law: Power, Duty, Constraint* and editor of *Public Health Law and Ethics: A Reader* (both University of California Press/Milbank Memorial Fund).

Mariëtte van den Hoven is Researcher/teacher at the Ethics Institute, Utrecht University; and Coordinator of the Netherlands Research School in Practical Philosophy. She wrote a PhD thesis on common sense morality and reasonableness, and has worked on numerous ethical issues in medicine and public health.

Jay A. Jacobson, MD, is Professor of Internal Medicine; Chief of the Division of Medical Ethics; and a member of the Division of Infectious Diseases at LDS Hospital and the Department of Medicine at the University of Utah School of Medicine. Current areas of interest and research include clinical and classroom teaching of medical ethics, infectious diseases, subspeciality consultation and patient care, end of life care, and informed consent and medical decision-making.

Bruce Jennings is Director of the Center for Humans and Nature in New York; and Senior Consultant at The Hastings Center in Garrison, NY. He also teaches at the Yale University School of Public Health. He is author of numerous books and articles on ethical and social issues in health care and public policy.

James O. Mason, MD, MPH, is an infectious disease specialist trained at the University of Utah who also holds an MPH from Harvard. He became Director of the National Centers for Disease Control and Prevention in 1983. He served as Executive Director for the Utah Department of Health and, in 1989, became head of the US Public Health Service.

Niels Nijsingh previously studied philosophy and is now a PhD student at the Ethics Institute at Utrecht University. His research concerns newborn screening programmes, informed consent, and paternalism.

Charles B. Smith, MD, is Professor Emeritus of Medicine at the University of Washington School of Medicine, having previously served there as Professor and Associate Dean. He served as Chief Medical Officer of the Veteran's Association Hospitals in both Salt Lake City and Seattle. He has held positions as Associate Chairman, Professor of Medicine, and Chief of the Division of Infectious Diseases, and is currently Professor Emeritus in the Department of Medicine at the University of Utah School of Medicine. Current research interests are in the field of medical ethics.

Tom Sorell is Professor of Philosophy at Essex University, UK. He has published extensively on Hobbes and Descartes, epistemology and philosophy of science, moral theory, and applied ethics. His many books include *Scientism* (1991) and *Moral Theory and Anomaly* (1999). He is currently working on a book project about emergencies and moral and political philosophy.

Lesley Stone, JD, is a Zuckerman Fellow at Harvard University's Kennedy School of Government. Previously, she was Senior Fellow at the Center for Law and Public's Health at Georgetown and Johns Hopkins Universities.

Marcel Verweij is Senior Researcher and Lecturer at the Ethics Institute, Utrecht University. He coordinates the international Masters programme in applied ethics. His main research interests are in public health ethics, notably vaccination programmes, screening, and infectious diseases control.

Daniel Wikler, PhD, is Mary B. Saltonstall Professor of Population Ethics in the Department of Population and International Health at the Harvard School of Public Health. He served as the first 'staff ethicist' at the World Health Organization in Geneva, working with WHO health programmes on ethical issues arising in departments throughout the organization, including health resource allocation, research involving human subjects, and genetics. While at WHO, Professor Wikler directed an international collaboration among philosophers and economists on ethical, methodological, and philosophical issues raised by WHO's work in measurement of the global burden of disease and in developing methods for improving health resource allocation.

His published work addresses many issues in bioethics, focusing in recent years on population health, including issues resource allocation, and global public health. His book series, *Studies in Philosophy and Health Policy*, was published by Cambridge University Press, as was *From Chance to Choice: Genetics and Justice*, co-authored by Prof. Wikler and three other philosophers.

PREFACE

The origins of this volume lie in conversations following the 5th World Congress of the International Association of Bioethics (IAB) in London in September 2000. It was at that event that we met and discovered a mutual interest in the ethical issues relating to public health. This joint interest has strengthened over the years through many joint research and teaching projects. Over the last five years we have discovered many others who share this interest, and we are very pleased to see that public health ethics is increasingly recognised as an important and growing sub-discipline. A significant influence upon this development has been the organisation of events at subsequent IAB world congresses and the work of the International Public Health Ethics Network (InterPHEN), a network of the International Association of Bioethics (IAB). We are grateful to the present and past members of the Board of the IAB for their support.

Some of these papers originate from a research seminar on the theme of Public Health and Ethical Theory held in Bilthoven in the Netherlands in May 2002 (co-sponsored by the Netherlands School for Research in Practical Philosophy and the Netherlands Organization for Scientific Research). Other papers are the result of later work from our friends and colleagues across the world. We are very grateful to all of the authors of the chapters in this collection for allowing us to publish their work and to join us in raising the profile of public health ethics.

Angus Dawson
Marcel Verweij

1

Introduction: Ethics, Prevention, and Public Health

Angus Dawson and Marcel Verweij

1.1. Aims of this Collection

Public health ethics is developing as a new sub-discipline within the broader field of bioethics. One important aim of this book is to strengthen this development by furthering existing discussions and stimulating new debates. The different chapters in this book cover a wide range of issues and theories related to public health: they refer to a diverse range of literature from many disciplines including philosophy, ethical theory, applied ethics, philosophy of science, political philosophy, medicine, public health, economics, and law. This diversity is a sign that public health ethics is (and needs to be) committed to interdisciplinary work. Each of the chapters has slightly differing aims, but a strength and theme of all chapters is that they draw upon both theoretical and applied work. It is not just that discussion of moral issues in public health requires the application of theory: reflection on such concrete problems can also in turn help to refine and develop more theoretical points of view.

In this introduction we have three main tasks. Firstly, we outline some core themes in public health ethics that are explored in the various chapters in this volume. Secondly, we situate the debates in these chapters in the existing public health ethics literature. Finally, we briefly outline the key points in each individual chapter.

1.2. Some Central Themes of this Book

Each of the individual chapters in this volume explores one or more concrete moral question in public health. In this section we pick out a number of themes that run through the following chapters. The first general theme is a focus on the idea of prevention. Public health practice and programmes that aim to prevent disease systematically raise moral concerns that are different from those in 'regular' health care practice. We begin this section by outlining three general features of preventive interventions. These features indicate key differences between public health and clinical medicine, but they also provide grounds for possible moral concern.

The first salient feature of preventive care and public health programmes is that the initiative usually comes from the public health professional, not the 'patient'. For example, in preventive programmes individuals are invited or encouraged to participate in screening programmes, to be vaccinated, or to change their 'unhealthy' behaviour: the request for such interventions does not come from the individual themselves. However, in health care practice, individuals generally visit a physician because they have experienced some sort of medical symptoms. Given the fact that public health programmes help people to avoid disease and are therefore paradigmatically targeted at healthy (or at least asymptomatic) people, target groups may need to be persuaded to participate. As long as persuasion is accomplished through disclosure of all relevant information, there will be few problems, but often the possibilities for extensive information disclosure will be limited. In other cases, varying degrees of coercion are employed in order to achieve successful participation rates in a programme. Personal autonomy, cherished in modern individual health care, might not be given priority in public health care, where other values, such as the protection of the health of individuals and groups, the prevention of harm to others, and the promotion of health equity, are central.

A second feature of public health is that, typically, interventions aim to protect and promote health at a group or population level. Successful programmes will aim to effectively reduce morbidity and mortality rates within a population at a reasonable cost (in terms of any expenditure and negative side-effects). Yet even though the benefits visible at the population level might easily outweigh the costs and possible harms, it may be perfectly reasonable for individuals to make a different evaluation of the costs and benefits for themselves as individuals. Some participants might see only potential inconveniences and burdens, and they might be uncertain as to whether the programme will be beneficial for them as individuals. This also happens in clinical medicine, of course, but then at least the treatment is intended to be beneficial for the individual patient. However, public health programmes may not be beneficial for each individual person, as there might well be a conflict between protecting the health of the public and the well-being of individuals. For example, quarantine procedures during the recent SARS outbreak in Toronto were not meant to protect the health of the quarantined persons themselves, but to protect the health of others in the population (Singer et al. 2003). The possibility of bioterrorist attacks with smallpox led to renewed smallpox vaccination programmes in the US, even though the vaccine is known to cause serious harm in some cases (Casey et al. 2006). Hence, public health interventions might turn out to be harmful to at least some individuals, and ethical reflection in public health will often involve discussion of this tension between public and private interests.

A third salient feature of preventive programmes (and many other public health activities) is their potential pervasiveness. Almost all things in life, one's lifestyle, the state of the social and physical environment, economic prosperity and environmental pollution, and all policies and decisions that are being made in these contexts, can have an impact on health. Public health aims to create a context in which people can live a healthy life, but this laudable objective might also provide a reason to meddle with almost all aspects affecting our lives. This raises ethical problems if public health interventions come to impact upon our ability to lead a life of our own, or if the pervasive public concerns for health would adversely impact upon our private lives and individual choices. One could also be concerned that a pervasive and continuous emphasis on the risks of disease and the promotion of health might lead to a neglect of other things of value, such as pleasure, courage, individuality, or being carefree (Verweij 1999). This capacity to prevent harm does not just concern each person's choices about their own health. Given our expanding medical and epidemiological knowledge we have more and more opportunities to avoid causing harm to others (through such things as second-hand smoke or increased risks of infection). This then raises the question of how far each person's responsibility for the health of others might extend.

In addition to these issues relating to prevention and health promotion, there are a number of other theoretical issues that are discussed in the chapters in this volume. One general theme is the extent to which the public good or the public interest might justify state interventions that impose limits upon the freedom of individuals. This problem is especially visible in infectious disease control, debates about water fluoridation, and some alcohol, drug and tobacco policies. For example, the recent control of the Severe Acute Respiratory Syndrome (SARS) outbreak in Asia and Canada in 2003 illustrates some of these issues. It provides an example that underscores both the importance of effective programmes to protect the public's health and the impact of such programmes upon community life and individual well-being. In this particular case both the relatively easy mode of transmission of SARS and the seriousness of the disease contribute to its significance as a public health problem. Such biological facts may be important in providing a justification for the stringent measures carried out with the aim of containing the spread of the disease. Even though the character of many of the public health measures undertaken to stop further spread of SARS in South East Asia and Canada may seem to date from earlier times—quarantine, isolation, and mandatory treatment—they may well be justified if the public at large is at real risk of a serious infectious disease. Treatment or preventive measures may be inconvenient, unwanted or even harmful for some individuals, yet such varying degrees of what is usually regarded as 'wrongness' may be considered an acceptable side-effect if they are genuinely necessary for protecting whole populations.

Whilst SARS has provided a focus for consideration of public health interventions and their justification, there are plenty of other urgent public health issues that require ethical exploration. For example, if current avian influenza virus strains mutate into an influenza virus that can spread from human to human, a new influenza pandemic might arise with immense morbidity and mortality rates. Pandemic preparedness action plans raise numerous ethical issues concerning isolation, quarantine, and allocation of scarce antiviral drugs and vaccines (Kotalik 2005). HIV infection rates continue to grow, leading to the death of millions of people throughout the world, and the slowing or even collapse of economic development in many nations (WHO 2005). During the last decades, tobacco use has been established as one of the most common causes of lung cancer and cardiovascular disease, but despite this its use in the developing world continues to grow (WHO 2004). And while public and political awareness of the risks of smoking are gradually increasing, at least in the developed world, obesity is presenting itself as a new 'lifestyle epidemic' (WHO 2000a).

The diverse efforts that are undertaken for protecting people's health against these risks are often extremely valuable, yet they raise numerous ethical concerns. In what cases, if any, is mandatory treatment justified? When should health care practices disclose medical information about individuals to public officials 'for the sake of public health'? Can parents be forced to accept vaccination of their children? Should unhealthy food products be banned? What interventions are justified to protect children against the tobacco smoke of their parents? Should governments actively aim to change people's preferences about such things as food, smoking, or physical exercise?

The imperative driving such policies in public health is perhaps strongest where action contributes to the creation or maintenance of a public good. What exactly public goods might be is a complex issue. However, they are certainly more than the mere aggregation of individual goods. This can be seen in the fact that once a public good is created, it cannot simply be broken down into individual goods. For example, once herd protection exists in a population, whilst individuals can choose not to participate in or to withdraw from a vaccination programme, they cannot withdraw from the benefit which they enjoy if herd protection exists in that population. Likewise, no one else can withdraw such a benefit from non-participating individuals. Public goods cannot be created by individuals or small groups of individuals. They generally require action on behalf of a sizeable part of a population, and this is why public health action is often carried out by governmental or quasi-governmental organisations. The capacity for such interference in people's lives, in the name of public health, has led to a great deal of discussion about the legitimate boundaries of state power and how the interests or rights of individuals can be preserved. Not all limitations to personal autonomy will be justified, just because there is a public interest at stake. The difficult issue is trying to determine what sort of conditions need to be satisfied for a freedom-limiting policy to be justified. Various chapters in this volume focus on this issue, using a number of different examples from public health practice. In an age in which medicine and health care have learned to see patient autonomy and the well-being of each individual as core values, public health programmes that limit freedom, impose treatment, and aim to adjust unhealthy behaviour might seem overly paternalistic or potentially coercive.

A related issue is to focus on the role of individuals in promoting public health. To what extent do individuals have moral obligations to contribute to protecting the community or the public good? This question is again highly relevant for many issues in public health, but is particularly important for policy in relation to infectious diseases and smoking. Some groups, like health care workers might be considered to have special obligations towards the public's health. Yet if we simply apply a popular principle from medical ethics, such as the suggestion that people should avoid inflicting harm upon others, this might impose very demanding requirements upon individuals. For example, it might imply an obligation to accept vaccination for the sake of preventing harm to others. Some will argue, using an appeal to recent debates on the demands of morality, that such an obligation would be *too* demanding. Such arguments draw upon recent criticisms of moral theories, particularly consequentialism. However, it would be a mistake to see this as only being a 'problem' for consequentialism as many theories are susceptible to the same objection. Even traditional forms of liberalism will invoke 'harm to others' as a justification for restricting the liberty of individuals in at least some cases.

Public health is therefore an interesting area for ethical discussion because it challenges us to think beyond the established consensus in much contemporary bioethics, and it brings us back to fundamental issues in moral theory and bioethics. It is not obvious that an appeal to simple principles such as the need to respect individual autonomy is going to provide a sufficient response to the complex issues we face when thinking about what is appropriate for populations as well as individuals. What sort of theoretical approach is most suitable to consider issues in public health? The chapters in this collection seek to extend the work that already exists in this field.

1.3. The Emerging Field of Public Health Ethics

During the last few decades the field of bioethics has developed with a special focus on moral problems relating to clinical encounters between patients and health care professionals. Yet the features of prevention and public health mentioned above indicate that ethical reflection in these areas will often be different from ethical reflection in other health care settings. In clinical ethics, the special nature of the professional–patient relationship is central, and many problems can be fruitfully analysed in terms of the obligations of the individual caregiver and the rights of the individual patient. Preventive interventions on the other hand, are often offered with a focus on populations and in such a way that individual health professionals fulfil a limited role within a larger organisation. These programmes are targeted at groups of people and aim to realise health benefits at a group or population level. Indeed, such public health interventions can be considered to be focused on *collectives* or groups, not just in terms of patients but also in terms of moral agents. In this way, the most common approaches in bioethics, focusing on decision making of individual professionals and their obligations towards individual patients, may be of limited use in clarifying and analysing moral problems in public health.

Until recently, few bioethicists seemed interested in writing about issues in public health. For example, the various editions of Beauchamp and Childress's key text *Principles of Biomedical Ethics* (1979, 2001), widely applauded as well as much criticised, have always focused on moral problems in care and cure. The focus on ethical issues at a group or population level—essential for understanding public health—is only apparent in discussions of justice in health care. Programmes for screening, vaccination, health promotion and education, the reduction of inequalities, and improvements to the environment through air, water and food control, though obvious parts of the field of biomedicine, receive no systematic discussion in such bioethics textbooks. Despite this relative neglect of public health in mainstream bioethics, there have always been some writers working on issues in public health and prevention. Good examples of excellent early work in these areas include work on smoking (Goodin 1989), paternalism and public health (Beauchamp 1976; Wikler 1978), responsibility for health (Wikler 1987) and health promotion (Downie et al. 1990). The diverse moral problems that were raised by AIDS and HIV prevention were discussed by a number of authors (Bayer 1991; Gostin and Lazzarini 1997; Bennett and Erin 1999; Gostin 2004b). Skrabanek (1990) criticised the lack of ethical discussion of preventive medicine in a famous paper published in the *Journal of Medical Ethics*. His critical comments were focused on 'ordinary' mass screening programmes—and not on the specific forms of screening that were most discussed by ethicists (antenatal screening and genetic screening programmes).

Over the last few years, however, things have gradually changed, and public health ethics has developed into a recognised branch of applied ethics (Beauchamp and Steinbock 1999). Topics such as infectious disease, the concept of prevention, immunisation policies, cancer screening, and drug and tobacco policies are being recognised as ethically relevant and interesting. Such themes are no longer the object of merely ad hoc ethical reflection, but are increasingly being discussed in a more systematic way (Buchanan 2000; Gostin 2000b; Verweij 2000). There are signs of a growing awareness of the many ethical issues that arise in public health and a growing number of publications reflect this. For example, a recent collection of original papers by Anand et al. (2004) explores issues relating to global health, equity and social justice. Cribb (2005) provides a sustained argument for considering ethical issues in bioethics from the perspective of the social context of health, and argues that this necessarily entails looking at medicine from the perspective of public health. Kessel (2006) has provided the first sustained discussion of ethical, historical, and public policy issues relating to air pollution. Other collections about to appear include recent work on the ethics of infectious disease (Selgelid et al. 2006) and public health ethics in general (Freeman forthcoming).

Increasingly, authors writing about public health are questioning the liberal political perspective that is common among many bioethicists and emphasising the need for a broader based approach when it comes to public health issues. This may mean working within a revised liberal approach, adapting a more traditional moral theory such as consequentialism or contractarianism, or adopting a more communitarian or republican justificatory framework for public health (Kass 2001; Callahan and Jennings 2002; Childress et al. 2002; Roberts and Reich 2002). This is an interesting example of how reflection upon particular issues can result in revisions at the more theoretical level. We will surely see interesting theoretical work in moral and political philosophy emerging in the future as a result of the discussion of public health practice.

1.4. Overview of this Book

Most of the chapters in this volume contribute to the discussion of the public or collective nature of public health. As argued above, public health measures might involve encroachment upon the interests of some individuals. Such infringements may sometimes be justified because the interests of the public as a whole are at stake. In Chapter 2, Marcel Verweij and Angus Dawson discuss various definitions of public health, and explore different possible conceptions of what might be meant by the concept of 'public' in the context of public health. They distinguish two main senses of 'public' at work in such definitions: public health as the *health of the public*, and public health as a set of *public or collective interventions* aiming at improving health. These two elements can be seen at work in some of the other chapters in this collection.

The political perspective on public health ethics is most strongly developed by Bruce Jennings in Chapter 3. His argument for a civic republican account of public health policy draws on a brief historical presentation of this set of political views. Civic republicanism seems a fruitful approach to public health, as it conceives members of the public as citizens. They are not just to be seen as the target for policies but as the central agents in the design and implementation of such policies. In this way, the two basic senses of 'public' in public health (as distinguished by Verweij and Dawson in Chapter 2) come together.

Effective public health protection cannot be realised without the implementation of and support of legal measures. Law plays an important role in regulating behaviour and directing people and institutions to contribute to health. Ethical questions arise most clearly in relation to public health interventions when they are compulsory and backed up by legal sanctions. Public health ethics is therefore intimately linked with public health law. Larry Gostin and Lesley Stone (Chapter 4) offer a rich understanding of public health law, and describe seven ways in which the law might be used as an active tool to promote the public's health.

In Chapter 5, Daniel Wikler and Dan Brock outline what they call 'population health'. This chapter briefly sketches some of the existing literature that has focused explicitly on looking at ethical issues from the population and global perspectives. The discussion considers some of the ethically relevant differences between policies that are directed at and organised within populations, and the actions of individuals towards each other. The chapter lays bare the work that still needs to be done in relation to these issues, and serves as an excellent starting point for anyone unable to see the need for work on ethical issues on the population level related to public health.

In Chapter 6, Tom Sorell uses resources drawn from the philosophy of science to argue that public policy should be shaped by a robust form of scientific realism. He argues that where clear evidence exists in favour of a policy, relevant experts broadly agree, and adequate consideration has been given to contrary public opinion, there is a moral obligation upon the public to accept these findings (and the subsequent policy). Sorell writes about concerns over the safety of the MMR vaccine, arguing that whilst parents' views are important, they should not have any 'extra' weight beyond the claims of public opinion already considered by the policy makers. He suggests that sometimes policy makers have a duty to stick by a policy based on the best available evidence despite the views of a vocal minority of the population.

One important instrument for evaluating public health programmes is cost-effectiveness analysis, in which health effects are measured in specific units (such as QALYs or healthy life years gained). Such tools enable comparisons to be made between different programmes and policies. The application of such quantitative methods as a tool for priority setting and political decision making is controversial. One complaint is that such methods focus on the aggregation of effects and ignore how such effects are distributed among (sub)groups. Dan Brock explores the value assumptions of cost-effectiveness methods as a tool for decision making in relation to vaccination programmes (Chapter 7). He argues that the issues of distribution and justice require separate discussion and that these aspects should not be incorporated in an adjusted model of cost-effectiveness.

Protection against infectious diseases seems to be one of the paradigmatic cases of public health. Three chapters discuss different issues with respect to such protection. In Chapter 8, Mariëtte van den Hoven focuses on a discussion of the obligations of individuals to contribute to the protection of others. She asks to what extent individuals in a specific context—health care workers in a nursing home—should contribute to the prevention of influenza. They might have obvious duties as health professionals towards their patients, but do such duties also imply an obligation to be vaccinated for the good of others? She discusses this case in the light of the recent theoretical debate about the limits of morality. Van den Hoven argues that in exploring the scope of moral obligation, we need to take account of the costs to the agent. She argues that if we do not, the moral obligations imposed through public health policies may be seen as unreasonably demanding.

In Chapter 9, Jay Jacobson et al. explore the morally salient dimensions of infectious disease by outlining and drawing attention to differences in present policy towards genetic and infectious disease. They use the contrasting cases of syphilis and cystic fibrosis to illustrate their argument. Jacobson et al. argue that despite the fact that in both cases the relevant diseases will potentially harm the parents' offspring, medical policy is significantly different relative to each case. They use this contrast to ask questions about the legitimate limits to paternalistic public health interventions.

One important reason for the promotion of vaccination against some infectious diseases is the possibility of creating and maintaining herd protection. If enough people within a group are immune, a contagious virus will have a reduced chance of reproducing and spreading among the members of the group. In this way the group as a whole is protected, even if some of the individual members of the group lack immunity themselves. In Chapter 10, Angus Dawson discusses the relevance of herd protection for arguments about our moral obligations to each other in relation to vaccination programmes. He argues that herd protection should be thought of an important public good, which we are all obligated to promote and protect. However, he argues that once herd protection exists in a population neither a harm-to-others argument nor free-rider considerations will be sufficient to generate such an obligation in relation to herd protection.

Marcel Verweij, in Chapter 11, focuses on a different branch of public health, namely tobacco discouragement programmes. Tobacco discouragement is controversial as it involves active government interference, not just in the behaviour of individuals, but also in aiming to change the preferences individuals have towards smoking. The aim of Verweij's chapter is to explore arguments relating to tobacco discouragement that avoid the easy charge of unjustified paternalism. He argues that utilitarian arguments might fail, unless they can make clear that tobacco discouragement is a public good that is not simply equivalent to the aggregation of the individual goods of the persons who are to be discouraged. Verweij argues that tobacco discouragement can indeed be seen in these terms.

Finally, in Chapter 12, Niels Nijsingh explores the practical and ethical problems in requiring an informed consent in the context of a dramatically expanded programme of newborn screening. He argues that whilst, at first, it might look tempting to require informed consent from parents, in reality this is likely to place too severe a burden on both the parents and society in general. This means that we are faced with a choice either to not implement technological developments in relation to the expansion of screening or to accept that we will need to find other means of protecting the interests of participants apart from informed consent. This takes us right back to one of the core issues in contemporary clinical bioethics. Indeed, one of the consequences of thinking about issues such as consent within the context of public health is that we may begin to reflect more critically upon such a consensus and revise our views more generally as a result.

2

The Meaning of 'Public' in 'Public Health'

Marcel Verweij and Angus Dawson

2.1. Introduction

'Public health' is a contested concept. It is presented and used in a variety of ways by public health practitioners, researchers and commentators. In this chapter we aim to do two things. The first is to outline and review existing definitions of 'public health' and offer brief comments on some of these proposed accounts. However, we will not offer and defend an alternative definition. Instead our second aim will be to focus on what might be meant by the term 'public' in an account of 'public health'. We suggest that there are two key elements that can be identified. We will distinguish them, and discuss each in turn. We argue that if we have a clearer idea of what is meant by 'public' in this context then perhaps we can make some progress in thinking through what 'public health' might be, and that this will in turn help us to provide a focus for exploring arguments about the moral justification of actions and inactions as part of a wider discussion of public health ethics.

We began with the suggestion that public health is a contested concept. Part of the reason for this fact is the way that the term 'public health' relates to the idea of a 'public health problem'. A great deal of effort goes into attempting to gain support for the idea that certain types of events or activities count as public health problems. For example, recent suggested candidates for the status of public health problems (to add to the paradigm cases of infectious diseases, smoking, pollution, inadequate sanitation, and societal inequalities) include domestic violence (Ramsay et al. 2002), teenage pregnancy (Scally 2002), gambling (Korn and Shaffner 1999), and suicide (US Public Health Service 1999). How are we to decide whether something is a legitimate candidate for public health activity? The answer to this question is that we need a clear and agreed characterisation of 'public health' itself. Some candidate definitions are discussed in the next section. However, we should note here that it is clear that something is gained by characterising a thing as a public health issue or problem. What might this be? There are a number of possible answers to such a question. It might be that by calling something a public health problem, attention is being draw to the fact that such events are common or increasing within a population (an epidemiological issue). Perhaps this designation emphasises the fact that such events are not solely dependent upon any individual agent's actions but are influenced to some extent by socio-economic and other background conditions (a causation issue). Perhaps the idea is that we should treat these issues in a particular way, possibly through collective or governmental rather than individual action (a responsibility issue). It might be that such events threaten important values in society and that this justifies particular forms of intervention (a polity issue). Or it might be that calling such things public health problems provides them with a particular emphasis or urgency, and that we are being asked to prioritise them, and see stopping them as an important moral issue (a normative issue).

There is no reason to think that these explanations are mutually exclusive or than any single one captures the complete story. However, given the diversity of aims and interests that may be involved in calling something a public health issue, we might expect the concept of public health to be indistinct as well. It is therefore no surprise that there is a wide range of definitions and descriptions of 'public health' in the literature. In the next section we consider some of these, as a first step in exploring the concept.

2.2. Definitions of 'Public Health'

In this section we outline a number of the most influential or interesting definitions or accounts of 'public health' available in the public health literature. This review is not supposed to be systematic or complete, but these accounts are chosen to enable us to pick out a number of different relevant features of public health to provide the basis for further discussion.

Public health is the science and the art of preventing disease, prolonging life and promoting physical health and efficiency through organised community efforts for the sanitation of the environment, the control of community infections, the education of the individual in principles of personal hygiene, the organisation of medical and nursing service for the early diagnosis and preventative treatment of disease, and the development of social machinery which will ensure to every individual in the community a standard of living adequate for the maintenance of health.

(Winslow 1920)

what we, as a society, do collectively to assure the conditions in which people can be healthy

(Institute of Medicine 1988)

the science and art of preventing disease, prolonging life and promoting health through organised efforts of society

(Acheson 1988)

'Government intervention as public health' involves public officials taking appropriate measures pursuant to specific legal authority . . . to protect the health of the public . . . The key element in public health is the role of the government—its power and obligation to invoke mandatory or coercive measures to eliminate a threat to the public's health.

(Rothstein 2002)

Society's obligation to assure the conditions for people's health

(Gostin 2001)

Childress et al. (2002) prefer to list 'features' or aspects of public health:

Public health is primarily concerned with the health of the entire population, rather the health of individuals. Its features include an emphasis on the promotion of health and the prevention of disease and disability; the collection and use of epidemiological data, population surveillance, and other forms of empirical quantative assessment; a recognition of the multidimensional nature of the determinants of health; and a focus on the complex interactions of many factors—biological, behavioral, social and environmental—in developing effective interventions.

The first thing to note is the diversity of these various definitions and accounts of 'public health'. Some offer what are clearly supposed to be *definitions* of 'public health', others present a list of features, characteristics or aspects of public health, without offering any core definition. Some of these accounts are very broad in their nature and scope whilst others focus on a more narrow range of considerations. Some are highly normative, whilst others are more or less descriptive. Some even contain detailed guidance as to how the relevant ends of public health are to be achieved. This multiplicity of concerns can be seen by looking at perhaps the most significant of all accounts of public health: that provided by Winslow (1920). His definition is clearly not just saying something about what public health is, but also contains some discussion about how public health is to be achieved and how things need to be arranged to bring these things about. Despite the fact that it was written in 1920, its influence can still be seen in many of the more recent accounts, such as those provided by Acheson (1988) and the Institute of Medicine (1988). In the rest of this section we will offer a framework to explore these various accounts in a systematic way. We begin with a distinction between what we call broad and narrow accounts of public health.

2.2.1. Broad and Narrow Accounts of 'Public Health'

There are different ways that a narrow−broad distinction can be drawn. The most important way is in relation to the issues to be covered by public health, that is, the *nature* of public health interventions. Should public health be defined narrowly, in a way that is strongly related to traditional conceptions of the field, or should a much broader definition be endorsed?[1] The 'traditional' approach would be to focus on the type of health factors mentioned in Winslow's definition: e.g. environmental factors, sanitation, infectious disease control, screening programmes, or health education. However, other writers want public health to be conceived as a much broader enterprise, dealing with all of the factors that might affect the health of people, including societal, cultural, and economic determinants of health (see Ashton and Seymour 1988). The main objection to narrow accounts of public health is that they fail to take into account many of the things that contribute towards public health problems. On this view, public health is primarily about prevention in its widest sense and true prevention will have to focus on all of the causes of public health problems. The challenge from the broad

---

[1] See the scheme in Gostin (2002b: 7).

account is that any other approach can just seem arbitrary, as no sound reason can be provided for focusing on the actual or chosen priorities for public health interventions in the narrow sense.

By contrast the broad accounts do not just focus public health attention on the 'traditional' elements of prevention, but expand their concern to pick out all factors that may influence health such as the socio-economic conditions of a society including issues like homelessness, violence, war, race, education, and wealth. All of these factors are held to be legitimate concerns for public health activity because they all impact upon people's health (in the broadest sense). Indeed, the aim of such an approach might be seen as the promotion of general societal well-being rather than the mere reduction or removal of specified threats to health in a narrow sense (such as direct risks to physiological functioning). In principle such a conception of public health could be limitless, as almost all human activities (and many inactivities) may affect health. Indeed, such 'broad' accounts end up being reminiscent of the WHO definition of health as: 'a state of complete physical, mental and social well-being' (WHO 1946). Whilst the influence of the WHO definition of health can perhaps be seen as a theoretical stimulus to such an approach, a more practical one is the fact that many public health practitioners explicitly see their role as advocates for the public's health as explicitly being a form of political activity.

However, such 'broad' definitions have a significant problem in that they are so inclusive, so packed with content, that they cease to have any clear focus or meaning (Griffiths and Hunter 1999: 1). If we employ such an approach, any intervention aiming at improving well-being is likely to count as a matter relevant to public health. The concept of 'public health', essentially, just collapses into that of generating well-being or welfare: as a result such a concept, arguably, loses any useful purpose. In other words, supporters of such broad accounts are likely to be caught by a dilemma. On the one hand, by calling something a public health problem underlines its importance, but, on the other hand, such a broad definition of public health seems to be almost without limits. Whilst, it might be impossible to avoid fuzzy edges to the concept of 'public health', any useful concept of 'public health' is going to have to be limited in some way.

There is also another way that a broad and narrow view of public health can be distinguished. In his paper, 'Rethinking the Nature of Public Health', Mark Rothstein (2002) argues against the *broad* view that public health is 'anything that affects the health of the community on [a] mass basis'. In contrast,

Rothstein argues for what he characterises as a narrow account focused on *government interventions* as the defining characteristic of public health. He suggests that the use of such authority is only justified if three conditions are met: firstly, where the health of the population is threatened by something (this will include environmental factors not just diseases); secondly, where the government has powers or expertise to meet that threat; and, thirdly, where the action of government will be more efficient or more likely to be beneficial than the actions of individuals. Rothstein's view might be criticised on the basis that he is not so much *defining* public health as seeking to establish the legitimate boundaries of (sometimes coercive) government intervention in people's lives for the purpose of promoting public health. Such concerns are clearly normative—so let's turn to our second distinction.

2.2.2. Descriptive and Normative Accounts of 'Public Health'

From an ethical perspective, there is an interesting difference between the definitions of Winslow (1920) and the Institute of Medicine (1988) on the one hand, and Acheson (1988) on the other. The latter definition seems more or less descriptive and normatively neutral. It is about social activities that aim to promote health. The former concepts, however, are at least partly normative in the sense that they ascribe particular responsibilities to the community, namely to realise a context in order to *assure* that people live in conditions that are *adequate* for the maintenance of health. This normative dimension is amplified by Lawrence Gostin when he defines public health as 'society's obligation to assure the conditions for people's health' (Gostin 2001). Such normative dimensions make clear why it is sometimes attractive to call particular problems a *public health* problem. Take the example of domestic violence (as mentioned earlier). If we acknowledge domestic violence as a public health problem then this might not only imply that we accept the possibility that the causes of such violence are public, in the sense of going beyond the behaviour and choices of the violent individuals, but that we also must agree that society as a whole has a *moral obligation* to do something about it.

This leads onto another important point about normativity. One advantage of including normative elements in such a definition is that, once we accept something as a suitable definition, we are compelled to accept it as being a guide for action. Calling something a public health issue seems to imply that it concerns us all and the focus, in all three of these definitions, is on a range of collective or societal activities that together contribute towards improved health and well-being. This aspect also seems to raise normative considerations in relation to our responsibility for such improvements. To what extent is it the responsibility of each individual to participate in public health activity? We will return to this issue in a later section, but for our purposes here we can just note that some definitions such as that provided by Rothstein see public health as linked to government action with the aim of public protection, even to the point of justifying restrictions upon the liberty of individuals in some circumstances. Indeed, certain types of public goods produced by collective or government action might only be brought about in this way, and cannot be established or maintained by individuals. Once again, this draws attention to the fact that the concept of 'public' seems to play an important role in normative argumentation about the legitimacy of public health activity. We will return to this point later.

However, there are some reasons to be cautious about a clearly normative definition of public health. Firstly, from an ethical point of view, it is important to ensure that normative aspects are as clear and explicit as possible. This might be a reason to aim at a separation between definitions of a subject matter on the one hand, and related moral principles on the other. For example, it might be important to distinguish the issue about whether a particular set of acts is to be considered a public health issue from that of whose responsibility it is to act in relation to them. Secondly, some might consider normative accounts of public health to be too political. This might mean that even those things we can all agree are public health issues get lost because of disputes about the more marginal cases. For example, whilst protection against infectious diseases (to give only one example) is a topic that is relevant for any political perspective, the question how far society or government should go in issuing protective public health measures is open to discussion. It would be ironic and dangerous if the public's health were threatened by the term 'public health' coming to be seen as presupposing a particular ideological perspective.

2.2.3. Conceptual Clarity and Necessary and Sufficient Conditions

Our discussion so far is not meant to imply that we are seeking to determine the correct limits of the concept of 'public health'. We are not interested in this chapter in attempting to determine the necessary and sufficient conditions for something to count as being a public health issue. Indeed, many of the more recent accounts of public health have wisely moved away from such a methodology. These accounts focus not on producing definitions but function through the production of lists of characteristics or elements rather than producing a traditional definition. For example, Childress et al. (2002) provide a list of 'features' or aspects of public health rather than a definition (as does Frenk 1992: 69). The account given by Childress et al. is particularly interesting as it includes not only an account of the aims of public health (a focus on the 'entire' population) and the 'determinants' of health, but it also includes a list of certain public health methodologies. Of course, it might be the case that public health uses different methodologies from those of traditional medicine. However, it is not clear that, as a result, we should include such aspects within any formulation of the definition of public health. It is no surprise that 'public health' is a difficult concept, if, as is the case, the concept 'health' is already understood in divergent ways. One can be sceptical about the possibility of developing definitions specifying necessary and sufficient conditions for the application of terms like 'health' or 'public health', but that does not rule out the use of either term. We can and do use them without much conceptual confusion.

In this section we have sketched some distinctions that might be useful in thinking about the different proposed definitions of public health. We have concluded that a useful definition of public health is likely to be a narrow one, and that at least some senses of 'public' involved in the discussion of public health seem to necessarily involve a normative aspect. Our discussion of various definitions of public health makes clear that there is a lot of conceptual disagreement, at least partly because there are a variety of different agendas at work when it comes to labelling something a 'public health' issue or problem. Yet simultaneously, we believe that there is a core content to the term that seems to be shared by most authors. In the next sections we aim to further clarify this core meaning of public health by focusing on the different meanings of the adjective 'public'.

2.3.   Two Senses of 'Public' in Public Health

Many of the varying definitions and concepts of public health seem to appeal to at least two common elements. Firstly, they almost all pick out interventions that aim at protecting and promoting the health of the public. Talking about the 'health of the public' obviously involves the health of more than one person (or even a few persons). Public health concerns the health of populations, or at least larger groups of persons. This explains why public health practice depends upon epidemiological evidence about morbidity and mortality figures relating to collections of individuals. Secondly, most definitions also assume that the interventions themselves are in some sense 'public': that is, they concern various types of collective action, often action by government or other public bodies. However, relatively little attention has been paid to developing a more precise description of what is meant by 'public' in public health. We believe that a better understanding of the term 'public', in the two senses of the health of the public and interventions by the public, might help to get a better grip on the concept of 'public health' itself.

To return to the main point of this section, 'public health' might then, equally, refer to two things—and this points at the dual role of the adjective 'public'. Firstly, starting with the health of individuals, it makes sense to talk about public health as the state of the health of the public; that is, the health of the population as whole, or a population's 'collective health' (Rose 1992: 63). This means that we can compare the public health of different populations or the same population over time. Secondly, in talking of 'public health' we often refer, not to the state of health of the public, but to a practice or a set of interventions aiming to protect the health of the public. The latter use is clear in most definitions, e.g. 'what we, as a society do . . .' or '. . . through organised community efforts'. These interventions are in some way organised either by public institutions or they are carried out through collective effort. Many public health activities are collective activities *par excellence* and would be impossible without cooperation between (groups of) individuals. In conclusion, we suggest that both the interventions and the objectives of public health are 'public' and go beyond the level of individuals. Taken as a whole, we propose that the practice of public health (roughly) consists of *collective interventions that aim to promote and protect the health of the public.* Whilst it is not our intention to add another definition to the many that have been discussed above, this very general description seems to fit with most prominent theories of public health, and moreover, it emphasises the dual way in which the idea of 'public' plays a role in public health. In the remaining two sections we say more about each of these two aspects of 'public'. We will first discuss the idea of 'the health of the public', and then analyse different ways in which public health interventions might be held to be 'collective' or 'public' interventions.

2.4. The Health of the Public

Talking about the health of the public is, in the first place, not just talking about the health of particular individuals. Much of our knowledge of health, epidemiology and medicine depends on data about large numbers: morbidity and mortality figures, life expectancy rates, in short, data about the health of the population at large. Such data also indicates the chance that a random person within the population will fall ill with some disease. However, it is important to see that this is different from a statement about that individual's own health. The public's health—or population health—is, in at least some sense, a sum (aggregate) of the health status of all members of the population. Public health interventions are expected to make a difference on a population level, and this seems to imply that they should affect the health of many. It might be unclear, even with hindsight, which persons *in fact* benefited from the intervention. This is one of the salient dimensions of prevention: effective primary prevention results in things that do *not* happen (e.g. the onset of disease in persons). For example, as a result of an effective Hepatitis B vaccination programme fewer people will get Hepatitis, yet the 'persons' that benefit are not identifiable, and success exists only in a statistical sense (through a comparison of the rates of disease prior to and following the programme). Without population health figures it would be impossible to give any evidence about the effectiveness of preventive interventions.

However, if we acknowledge that public health interventions aim at improving the health of the population rather than of individuals, we should make three qualifications. Each qualification helps to get a better understanding—although also a more complicated picture—of what is meant by 'the public's health'. The first concerns the problem that population health is meaningless without reference to the health of individuals. After all, population health is (at least) dependent on the health of all individuals in the population, as it is, in some sense the sum, or the aggregate, of the health of all the relevant individuals. Assuming this dependence, the statement that particular interventions aim at the health of the public rather than at individual health seems to imply that such interventions should be successful enough so that any effects are visible at the population level. In other words: they should promote health on such a scale that it is visible in aggregate population health figures.

However, this aggregative picture does not completely cover our concept of the public's health, and this leads onto our second qualification. Suppose there are two populations in which the average life expectancy is exactly the same. The only difference concerns how mortality figures are 'distributed' within each population. In the first population it appears that each person has a more or less equal chance of enjoying a long life. In the second population, it appears that, on average, people living in a particular region, and also people with a very low income, live much shorter lives than people in other groups. In such a case, it is reasonable to think that the public health of the first population is higher than in the second. If this is true, then the concept of 'the public's health' does not only involve aggregation of the health of all constituent individuals, but it also has a distributive dimension.

Finally, there is an important sense of 'public health' that is not captured by the aggregative dimension or by the distributive dimension. This leads onto our third and final qualification. Many interventions might improve the public health even if their effects would remain invisible in both the aggregative and distributive health figures. For example, a community in which everyone is keen to avoid risks of transmission of infectious diseases, and where safer sex is a 'normal' practice, could be said to have a stronger public health than a community that lacks such attitudes; even though, luckily, both remain equally free from large outbreaks of the relevant disease. This points to an important dimension of public health that cannot be reduced to the aggregative or distributive aspects of the concept, and suggests that the state of the 'public's health' consists of more than the aggregative and distributive health figures referred to above. For example, an important part of our concept of public health refers to the underlying determinants of disease, notably the causes that are 'shared' among the public, and the extent to which such causes are contained, controlled or excluded from the population. An illustration of this point is provided by Lalonde's famous model of disease determinants, where the societal and environmental determinants are seen as being important dimensions of public health (Lalonde 1974). Our social practices as well as our social and physical environment are important determinants of the health of all members of the public. These environmental factors in the widest sense of the term encompass risks (and also health enhancing factors) that are in a sense 'open to all'. A society in which such health risks are relatively well contained, and in which health enhancing factors are well developed, can be said to have a stronger public health compared to other societies (other things being equal).

This last dimension of 'public health' has a strong connection with our basic understanding of the concept of 'the public', in the sense of the difference between talking about the public (or the public interest) as being different from a well-defined group of specified individuals (and their individual aggregated interests). As we saw above, there is a sense in which 'the public' refers to an indefinite number of non-assignable individuals, as Jeremy Bentham amongst others has suggested (Barry 1965: 229; Bentham 1996). The 'public' in this sense might refer to all members of a given community or state, but it need not, as a 'public' can also involve a smaller group of persons, as long as the persons are not specified. For example, in the context of a public health response to prostitution, all actual clients (and all persons who would consider visiting a prostitute) are members of the relevant 'public'. Improving the underlying social and environmental conditions of health will affect the health of persons, and that is an important reason for action, even though it will often be impossible to determine who exactly benefited from it. That the 'public' in public health refers to an *indefinite number* of individuals does not mean that any improvement in relation to public health necessarily implies improvement of the health of *many* persons. The number cannot be specified. For example, improving protection against a bioterrorist attack might save millions of people, or it might save 'only' a few. But the important thing is that it might be any one of us, who is saved. Any individual member of the relevant community has a share in the benefit from the improvement in public health. Similarly, in economic and political theory, public goods are goods that are open to all: it is not specified in advance which particular individuals will benefit from those goods. However, whilst such goods are 'open to all', this does not necessarily imply that every person will indeed benefit. On the other hand, just because any individual benefits are 'merely' statistical does not mean that the intervention is unethical. However, it does mean that we should think clearly about whether or not it is justifiable, preferably, before it is introduced.

To conclude, talking about public health in the sense of 'the health of the public' has several dimensions. First, it may refer to the sum of the health of all individuals in the relevant group or population. Second it might also refer to the way that health is 'distributed' in a population. And finally, an important sense of public health refers to underlying social and environmental conditions that might affect the health of each member of the public.

2.5. Collective Interventions

In its second role in public health, the term 'public' refers to a specific sort of practice, intervention, or policy that is aiming at population health through collective means. Again, the basic idea is that public health interventions are not primarily actions of individual persons, but they involve some form of collective action. One straightforward understanding of this is to say that these interventions are always (or perhaps, normally) *government* interventions. After all, government is the ultimate public body, and normally we assume that public institutions are in some way linked to government. As we have seen some authors, such as Rothstein, and perhaps less strictly, Gostin, restrict the field of public health to policies or interventions by government.

However, it is also possible that programmes that aim to improve the public's health are developed by private (or at least non-governmental) institutions. For example, originally, vaccination programmes in the Netherlands were carried out by societies of which anyone could become a member, some of the sanitary improvements of the nineteenth century in the UK were carried out by private water companies, and a great deal of international public health work is carried out by inter-governmental organisations such as the World Health Organization. Vaccination or screening can also be offered by individual physicians or within the context of employment. In all such cases this can still be considered a collective action if such activities fit within an overall programme in which many people cooperate in order to realise objectives that go beyond improving the health of assignable individuals. Arguably, most objectives with respect to improving the public's health (in any of the senses discussed above) cannot be realised by one person, acting on his or her own. To improve average health, to reduce health inequalities, or to improve those conditions that are relevant for the health of anyone, will normally require joint and coordinated action by many people and institutions. Governments will often play an important role in facilitating or coordinating these efforts, although this might not always be necessary.

There is also another important sense in which public health efforts are collective efforts: that is that, to be successful, public health interventions often require the active participation of members of the public. There are three ways that individuals might participate. Firstly, many health protection efforts can be left to specialist individuals or institutions, such as the organisation of a sewage systems, food safety control, infectious diseases control, etc. (One might of course argue that citizens do participate in such programmes through their tax payments). However, many other preventive interventions require the participation of individual citizens, for example: vaccination programmes, mass screening, safer sex campaigns, and other forms of health information and education. Some of these public health activities involve the participation of individuals to ensure the protection of *any one of us*; hence they are public issues *par excellence*. Examples are not drinking and driving; not smoking at the workplace; and practicing safer sex.

Secondly, other public health interventions involve participation by individuals in which each person takes care of their own health, for example: following recommendations about exercise, smoking reduction, or a healthy diet, or participating in cancer screening programmes.

Thirdly, and finally, sometimes the participation of individuals is not just important for those individuals themselves, but it is necessary because their *joint* participation itself might contribute to *public* health, in that it will improve the conditions for good health for all. High participation rates in vaccination programmes might lead to herd protection or even eradication of disease, to the benefit of all. Collective efforts to reduce smoking might make it easier for anyone to stop smoking or ensure that fewer people start to smoke. Such an approach might appeal to the idea of public goods as a means of justifying such collective action. This idea in turn might be linked to the idea of the 'background conditions' for the public's health, as discussed in some of the definitions of public health we considered above.[2]

---

[2] See, for example, the Institute of Medicine's (1988) definition.

These conditions are the things that no individual can do anything about on their own. One important consequence of such public goods is that collective action can create benefits that are open to all, indeed, even to those who do not contribute to the generation and maintenance of such goods.[3] This third type of participation also shows a link between our two senses of 'public', as it might well be here that our moral obligations to others, and arguments for government intervention, even to the point of restrictions upon our individual liberties, are strongest. Where there are public health benefits for the public as a group, which can only be obtained through collective rather than individual endeavour, public health action is most clearly justified. This is and should be the core of public health.[4]

Of the three ways in which the participation of the public is needed, the first and third are most clearly related to the *public* dimension of public health. In these two types of examples we might also have reason to think that members of the public most obviously have some sort of obligation to participate as individuals. With respect to the first category this obligation can be grounded in the general principle that citizens should refrain from harming each other. With respect to the third category, one could argue that citizens have some obligation (based on reciprocity or fairness) to contribute to a common good. Whether or not there is indeed a case for obligations to contribute to public health will, arguably, depend on the magnitude of both the risks and the goods that can be attained. Such a discussion however goes beyond the scope of this chapter. All three ways invoke public health in terms of activities but the second category might be considered to be less obviously part of the core of public health. However, even where the emphasis is upon the individual's action in relation to their own body and health, there are clearly relevant public health considerations, most obviously to do with health promotion and the availability of information and advice.

2.6. Demarcating the Area of Public Health?

One reason for seeking clarification of the meanings of 'public' in relation to the concept of 'public health' is to gain some grip on the subject matter

---

[3] See Chapter 1 and Chapters 10 and 11 by Dawson and Verweij in this volume for further discussion of the idea of public goods and public health.

[4] Many of the chapters in this volume explore examples of such public health activities.

of public health, so that discussion of public health issues can be isolated from other related issues, if only to make discussion possible. For example, clarifying the concept of public health may help to demarcate the area of public health (and distinguish it from medicine) as well as the area of public health ethics (and distinguish it from medical ethics). However, it is important not to be over precise in such differentiation because there are at least some interventions that seem to be part of both practices and so it is no surprise that there is a large overlap between medical ethics and public health ethics. If we were to accept that the two fields emphasise different values (e.g. medical ethics focuses on individual health and autonomy, and public health ethics concentrates on the common good) this might lead to confusion when it comes to the analysis of any moral issues that arise within any overlap between the two areas of medicine and public health. This would be the case even if we were willing to accept the hypothesis that there was no overlap between the values applicable in both areas of concern. In our view it does not make sense to 'clarify' such issues by drawing a sharp line between these two fields. On the contrary, many issues will almost certainly require reflection on how to balance different and possibly conflicting values from 'both' areas.

However, having said this, sometimes the assessment of the ethical issues will differ depending upon whether the intervention is considered to be a public health intervention or not. For example, some years ago, a programme for hepatitis B vaccination among 'high risk groups' was developed in the Netherlands (Heijnen et al. 2004). One of the central questions for the programme was whether the programme should be considered a public health intervention or as a form of preventive medical care for those individuals at risk. This was considered to be an important issue with respect to a number of decisions about the nature of the programme. For example, this concern could be seen in the discussion about whether it was necessary to offer all participants post-vaccination blood tests, in order to see if they showed a sufficient immune response to the vaccine. The rationale would be that low-responders could then be offered an extra series of vaccinations to increase their immunity. After discussion, the committee who prepared the implementation plan agreed that the programme should be considered a *public health programme*, and not primarily as a form of preventive care aimed at those individuals at risk. If the aim is to reduce transmission within a risk group, it might be acceptable that a few participants will be insufficiently protected. On the other hand, if the principal aim was to provide at-risk individuals with preventive care (i.e. immunity against Hepatitis B) there would have been stronger reasons to test whether the goal (sufficient immune response) has indeed been realised in each individual. In such a situation it might even be argued that it would have been unethical to refrain from post-vaccination testing.

However, in response to such debates, it seems to us that it might be more helpful to specify the goals of an intervention, consider which means are possible, and then determine which of the means available may be most justifiable in attempting to attain that goal. It is not clear that anything is to be gained by having an abstract discussion about whether a programme is *either* a public health intervention *or* a form of preventive medical care. Clearly if the medical/public health distinction is taken too seriously we run the risk of merely re-describing any programme to ensure that it is judged according to the viewer's perception of its moral legitimacy or, more practically, according to where sources of funding for such a programme might be found.

2.7. Conclusion

In this chapter we have explored some of the existing definitions of public health, but have not sought to develop a new definition of our own. However, we hope that the distinctions we have drawn and the discussion of the two senses of 'public' begin to help make clear what things might really be at the heart of public health. Calling something a public health problem often serves implicit normative or political purposes. This provides grounds for caution in thinking about the concept of 'public health' and public health activity. In ethical reflection, normative arguments and value statements should be made explicit, not disguised in seemingly descriptive terms. Let's return to the example of domestic violence again. It is certainly an individual tragedy for everyone involved; and we should certainly do all we can to reduce it, both as individuals and as a society. However, we are not dismissing it as an issue if we suggest that it is not really clear that domestic violence should be considered primarily the responsibility of public health officials, or if we ask what is added by calling it a *public health* problem.

3

Public Health and Civic Republicanism: Toward an Alternative Framework for Public Health Ethics

Bruce Jennings

'Ah, I see now!' Rambert exclaimed. 'You'll soon be talking about the interests of the general public. But public welfare is merely the sum total of the private welfares of each of us.'

The doctor seemed abruptly to come out of a dream.

'Oh, come!' he said. 'There's that, but there's much more to it than that . . .'

(Albert Camus, *The Plague*)

3.1. Introduction

In order to reduce disease and promote health, public health must be an agent of change—behavioral change among individuals and institutional change in societies. Change is never politically easy, or morally straightforward.

Existing patterns of behavior and institutions are embedded in structures of power and in discourses of legitimation. This is true at both the societal and the personal level, and change at either level requires normative justification. In truth, the requirements of normative justification are quite demanding in the arena of public health because changes of the magnitude required usually involve some form of state action—the creation of legal sanctions and enforcement, the creation of administrative structures, the investment and allocation of resources, and the mobilization of popular support.

During the life-time of modern public health in the industrialized West (roughly the past two centuries), the predominant framework of normative justification for state action has been provided by the tradition of philosophical liberalism. Within that broad stream there are several tributaries that have provided guidance and support to public health efforts. These include a form of natural rights contractarianism, economic and civil libertarianism, and utilitarianism or welfarist liberalism. Most recently one must add the international human rights framework, which, while certainly global in scope and meaning today, can be said to have its roots in the liberal traditions of the political cultures of Western Europe and the North Atlantic (Jennings 2003a).

It is not surprising then that public health ethics should show itself to be predominantly a child of liberalism. The language of policy justification that liberalism offers public health is primarily a language of rights, liberties, obligations, and autonomy on the contractarian and libertarian side; and a language of interests, utilities, preferences, and beneficence on the utilitarian or welfarist side. Liberty-limiting state actions are subject to a calculus of risk–benefit ratios, means–end rationality, and the balancing of individual rights of self-determination with obligations of self-restraint. The autonomy and respect due to adult individuals is pitted against the prevention of harm to self and others and the maximization of net benefit across a population.

Liberalism offers a serious agenda of issues for public health ethics, to be sure. Nonetheless, as in Rambert's appeal to private interests, something important is missing in this agenda. In this chapter I propose to explore the way public health ethics and practice have been situated within the liberal tradition, and the limitations this imposes on public health's moral discourse. The liberal framing of public health ethics is useful up to a point, but it is ultimately too narrow to provide normative justification for—or adequate moral insight about—the kinds of social change public health must strive to bring about.

To that end, I take up four topics:

1. Why does public health ethics need to go beyond liberalism?
2. To what extent can important conceptual resources for public health ethics be found in the tradition of civic republicanism in political theory?
3. How should the concept of civic virtue figure in public health ethics, and how should it be understood? And
4. what concepts of the 'public' or the 'common good' are available to public health ethics and which of them are most serviceable for public health ethics today?

3.2. The Limits of Liberalism for Public Health Ethics

Why does public health need a second ethical language to supplement liberalism, and where is that going to come from? To take up a second language of moral discourse is not unlike becoming fluent in a second natural language. What is involved is a gestalt shift in perception, and a paradigm shift in moral sensibility or imagination. The limits of our sense of moral possibility are called into question, as are the limits of what we regard as socially necessary or 'natural.' The horizon of moral responsibility also shifts. What I have in mind is closely related to what C. Wright Mills referred to as the difference between seeing a social problem as a 'personal trouble' and seeing it as a 'public issue.' Our scientific or descriptive analysis of where a problem comes from and what can be done about it changes. But so does our moral perception of how serious it is for the society as a whole, and who is responsible for doing something about it. Mills linked the ability to make this shift of perspective to the effects of the critical study of sociology (or the social sciences more generally), what he called 'the sociological imagination.'[1]

---

[1] Mills (1959). What Mills has in mind here should not be confused with another distinction, which is a staple of the liberal tradition, namely the distinction between the public and the private. A zone of privacy (both in the sense of control over personal information and personal freedom and discretion) is not incompatible with seeing experiences as social issues rather than as personal troubles. Indeed, when privacy is unjustly and unduly violated, it is precisely the ability to see this state of affairs as a social problem and not merely as a private trouble that makes it politically possible to resist such violation. Mills is talking about ideological distortions that reduce social

There are several reasons why this perspectival shift and this exercise of moral imagination are necessary to the future of public health ethics. Some of them have to do with the mission and political situation of the field of public health. Others have to do with conceptual and philosophical limitations that are prevalent, I would say inherent, in the liberal tradition.

3.2.1. Public Health as a Civic Profession

I regard public health as belonging to a cluster of disciplines and practices that might be referred to, for want of a better term, as the professions of public service or the 'civic professions.' These fields or professions include public administration, policy analysis, planning (urban, environmental, land-use planning, and the like), the military and law enforcement or public safety fields (police and fire protection), some aspects of the fields of education, communication, architecture, and law. Writers, academics, and teachers who are sometimes referred to as public scholars, public intellectuals, and social critics would be included as well (Schön 1983; Friedmann 1987; Jacoby 1987; Walzer 1987; Forester, 1989, 1999). These are the experts to whom we turn for their civic intelligence, leadership, and problem-solving capacity.

Even in an ideal democracy (one more egalitarian, participatory, and deliberative than any current polity), such civic or public service professions would be essential components of a vibrant political culture and state institutional apparatus. In the far less democratic systems of parliamentarian, presidential, and constitutional government that we do have, we entrust these civil servants and professionals with a large measure of stewardship over the common good. We rely on them to educate and enlighten us about what the common good consists in and what social justice requires in a practical, programmatic sense. We look to these professionals to transform power into authority and to provide us with the good reasons that will persuade us to voluntarily comply with all manner of rules, regulations, and recommendations that are conducive to life together and to our own best interests.

If confined to a liberal ethical language focused on individual rights, liberties, interests, and utilities, public health will not be able to fully grasp its distinctive vocation as a profession of public service. Moreover, it will not

and political phenomenon to individualistic terms; he is not prescribing that there should be no boundary line between public and private, nor even where that line should be drawn.

be able to deal adequately with the health needs and realities it must address through authoritative and legitimate public policy. In the face of infectious disease threats, public health will have to find an argument robust enough to justify coercion and paternalism. Those infected who directly spread disease may have their liberty curtailed on standard liberal grounds by appeal of the harm principle.[2] But public health measures must go beyond infected individuals and interfere with the lives of those not yet infected—limiting their movements, quarantining and destroying their property—and restricting their freedom and interests in many other ways. Such measures are not plausibly justified by appeal to the harm principle put in the future conditional tense. ('If you become infected you may harm others, so we will prevent you from being at risk of infection.') A more straight forward justification involves appeal to the notion of limiting and preventing the further spread of infection as itself an ethically worthwhile objective, a common good.

Or, to take another example, in the face of an aging society marked by chronic illness and life-style related risk factors, public health will have to work by means of persuasion rather than coercion (Jennings 2003a). Public health will have to engage with people at the grassroots level about the very difficult questions of what is human flourishing and what does it mean to live well as one ages with chronic disease. Such conversations will need to be richer than the language of interests and the right to be let alone.

Finally, as we learn more about how individual health risks are related to the context within which one lives one's life and makes health-related choices, the more we learn that the norms, networks, and institutions (so-called 'social capital') that comprise community are themselves an important determinant of health for individuals and communities. (Putnam 1995, 2000; Wilkinson 1996; Baron et al. 2000). In this case too, public health officials will need to speak a language of civic responsibility, engagement, and care in order to tend the fabric of institutions and relationships in civil society that keep people healthier throughout their lives.[3]

The language of liberalism forces public health professionals to appeal to 'interests' when the issue really does not have to do fundamentally with

---

[2] The harm principle states that the exercise of individual liberty that harms others without their consent may be curtailed by the state (see Feinberg 1973).

[3] For another view, and an interesting attempt to fashion a moral language to meet this challenge out of the resources of contemporary liberalism, particularly the work of Rawls, see Daniels et al. (1999).

individual needs and desires. It leads one to argue in terms of the promotion or restraint of autonomy when the issue isn't one of choice, but one of comparing an entire form of life with other possible ways of living. It leads one to talk of preference when the question is one of discernment and judgment. It leads one to talk of utility and welfare when the question is one of distinguishing between those relationships that are merely instrumental to the human good and those that are constitutive of it.

3.2.2. Conceptual Limitations of Liberalism

The gap between liberal concepts and the richer moral meaning that public health professionals often need to convey in justifying policies is a symptom of the enduring individualism of the social ontology and the moral psychology we inherit from the liberal tradition. Liberalism as a whole is fundamentally an individualistic ethical, epistemological, and ontological orientation, although different strands of the tradition, such as contractarianism and utilitarianism, are individualistic in different ways.[4]

There are times when public health problems and proposed solutions to them are not comprehensible or articulatable unless one has recourse to the concept of a public thing (*res publica*). But this is a sophisticated concept. How best to render it?—a social whole, a collective phenomenon, a shared, or common condition of life?

Many in the field seem to believe that the subject matter, methods, and technical expertise of the field provide adequate conceptions of what is public: we deal with the health of populations, we deal with large statistical samples, we deal with patterns of disease in different populations across time—all this is just what it means to study *public* health.

This won't quite do. Granted, health and disease are different when looked at from a population perspective than when looked at clinically or from the

---

[4] For contractarianism, the natural human individual prior to society is the basic unit of ethical and political value. The life, liberty, and happiness (if one is Jeffersonian) or property (if one is Lockean) of such an individual are the baseline of ethics. For the utilitarian orientation, it is the happiness of the greater number, not the individual, that provides the foundation for morality. However, neither Bentham nor any of his followers posited independent being or ontological status to that entity, the 'greater number'; only human individuals are the real beings in their metaphysics as in Locke's (Halévy 1966). Therefore the basis for ethics in utilitarianism is individuals in the aggregate; or to put it slightly differently, it is the aggregation of multiple separate states of individual happiness.

perspective of an individual. But if it is populations we study, it is the public we should serve. I maintain that the public is not a statistical concept, and it is not an aggregation of individuals. A 'public' is a community of individuals intertwined through complicated institutional and cultural systems in (and through) which they act and carry out their lives. Moreover, the public is not simply a descriptive concept—it is not just any configuration or system of interrelationship and life in common—it is a normative concept that provides an account of how that system should be structured and how our lives in common ought to be composed and lived. When a profession of public service (including public health), serves the public, it serves not only the public as it may be in the present, but it also serves an emergent, imaginatively corrected public.[5] Public health serves health today so as to promote the becoming of a potential public of greater justice and human flourishing tomorrow.

In a tangential way, public health is already thoroughly familiar with the problem of conceiving of object of study that are not comprehensible as aggregation of individual things. Consider a 'system'—a complex network of interacting and interrelated component elements—that has properties no one of its individual components possesses on its own. Or, again, consider the special mathematical properties of statistics and probability theory, and the special use of statistics employed in epidemiology in the service of public health. These intellectual tools indicate that simplistic notions of populations as aggregates of atomistic elements are inadequate to the *science* of public health. There is no reason why we should not recognize that these conceptions are also too simplistic for the *ethics* of public health. Public health needs more than the individualistic thinking inherent in the liberal tradition.

Another reason public health must go beyond individualistic thinking has to do with the kinds of human situations and behaviors that are related to health and disease. Human acts are intentional, purposive and meaningful both to the actors and to others who share in the rule-governed forms of

---

[5] It is worth clarifying here that there is a difference between the notion of the emergent and the notion of emerging. An emerging public is one that develops diachronically, across time via some process of social learning or becoming. What I have in mind here is the more synchronic notion of how the same people in the same generation can come to see themselves and their situation differently, sometimes quite abruptly and suddenly. The point here does not have to do with intergenerational justice, although that is clearly an important topic for public health ethics, but with the fact that greater democracy or an enriched moral sensibility are latent possibilities possessed by contemporary societies.

life and communication within a society and culture. The ethical norms that fit into human agency therefore are not limited to self-referential states of interest or desire. In order to understand ethical conduct—or in order to engage in ethical discourses of justification and other forms of argument—one must have recourse to concepts and categories that reflect the relational nature of the human self or actor and the contextual, social nature of the actor's meaningful, symbolically mediated relationships with others (Harré 1998).

Public health must strive to bring about change at both the level of individual behavior and social norms and institutions. But the individual level in question is already thoroughly social and relational in character, and change at the social level, in the final analysis, is nothing other than a change in the ways in which individuals experience and live their own social being.

In practice this means that for public health to respond to the coming health needs of complex societies, it must have recourse to values and purposes that the members of these societies will understand if they think and act like 'citizens' in the classic sense (irregardless of their legal or immigrant status) by coming to see private troubles as public problems. Public health professionals must be civic educators. Public health must identify and interpret for society changes in patterns of disease and risk that are not analytically reducible to individual behavior, but have systemic properties that come from structures of interpersonal relationships. Public health must incorporate into its moral discourse concepts of the right and the good that pertain not to individuals in isolation but to selves-in-relationships; not atomistic bearers of interest, preference, and desire but social persons whose personal flourishing is inextricably linked to the flourishing of others. In addition to the liberal language of rights, interests, and utilities, public health ethics needs the vocabulary of solidarity, mutuality, interdependency, social justice, community, and the common good. Beyond the notion of moral obligations that are correlative to the rights and interests of others, public health needs to appeal to a motivational structure that is informed by what has been traditionally called 'civic virtue.'

Is there a tradition of ethics and political theory that public health can turn to in order to find conceptual resources that are not readily available in the liberal tradition? In point of fact, there is a historically available tradition where many of the concepts and categories needed today by public health were once common currency. That tradition is now generally referred to by historians as 'civic republicanism' or 'civic humanism.' The next section sketches in broad strokes the intellectual history of republican political theory. I believe it would be beneficial for scholars and practitioners of public health to become more conversant with the history of political thought generally and thus have attempted to provide this background. Following this historical excursus, I return to conceptual analysis in Section 3.4.

3.3. A Sketch of Civic Republicanism

Civic republicanism was a central language of political thought in Europe, England, and the English-speaking colonies in North America from roughly the sixteenth century until the mid-nineteenth century, when it was supplanted by modern versions of liberalism, socialism, and communism. During the last thirty years republicanism has found renewed interest among political and intellectual historians. It has also enjoyed some revival among contemporary political theorists, usually in conjunction with their critiques of mainstream liberalism or utilitarianism and in tandem with the rise of a school of political theory generally referred to as 'communitarianism.'[6] This is not the place to attempt either a full intellectual history of republicanism or a critical assessment of its legacy and current importance. I hope instead to provide enough background to launch a discussion of the use of republican concepts in contemporary public health ethics.

The intellectual father of civic republicanism or civic humanism was Machiavelli. He, together with other historians and political thinkers active in the Italian city states of the renaissance, built civic republicanism on a revival of interest in the work of classical Greek and Roman thinkers, in particular the political writings of Aristotle, Cicero, and other Roman philosophers during the period of the republic, as well as the work of later Roman historians such as Livy and Polybius.

---

[6] I should point out that this has little to do with the ideology of the American political party that bears the same name. Contemporary political theorists who come to mind as drawing on civic republicanism in important ways include, Michael Sandel (1984), Benjamin Barber (1973), Quentin Skinner (1997), Charles Taylor (1985), William M. Sullivan (1982), Cass L. Sunstein (1993), and Philip Pettit (1997). And although her work is impossible to classify, one must include of Hannah Arendt (1973) in the story of the contemporary revival of republicanism.

Civic republicanism offered a vision of an ideal state of political life and political institutions. This vision was not 'democratic' in the contemporary sense of the term, but it was much more popularly based and participatory than the prevailing model of absolute rule found in late medieval writings on natural law, which underpinned the monarchies and principalities of the early modern period. Republicanism included a notion of a free people in a highly unified and patriotic political culture of civic service and responsibility. The republican notion of liberty or freedom provides an alternative to the liberal conception of liberty, which has been so influentially explicated by Isaiah Berlin, in his famous distinction between negative and positive liberty.[7] Republican liberty is a form of communal and social living from which arbitrary power and domination are absent. (Pettit 1997; Skinner 1997) This notion shares with the liberal tradition the importance of protecting or liberating the individual from being used as an object or an instrument of the rich, powerful, or those in political authority. But it defends this notion of liberty without holding that the individual must be seen atomistically. Individuals, like states, are relational beings, and they may be justly held to certain behaviors by proper authority in so far as that authority is not arbitrary from a moral point of view, and the relationships are not modes of domination. Notions of equity, reciprocity, mutuality, solidarity, and balance are central to the republican understanding of what constitutes a morally acceptable relationship, and what does not.

Underlying social and class conflicts were ever present in the minds of republican theorists, but these conflicts could be controlled and kept in check, according to many in this tradition, by a mixed form of government. This mixed and moderate political form was called—drawing on terminology borrowed from Aristotle (*politeia*) and from Roman thinkers (*res publica*)—a 'republic,' and was set in contrast to the other possible forms of government that reflect rule by the dominant class, namely monarchy, oligarchy, and democracy. Each of these forms was seen as prone to stifle free civic life in favor of the vested interests of the dominant group. To avoid this, republics were to have institutions that blend monarchical, aristocratic, and democratic elements.

---

[7] See Berlin (1969) and Skinner (1997). Skinner argues that the republican concept of freedom as the absence of arbitrary power and constraint provides both an alternative and a morally and politically attractive synthesis of what Berlin had identified as negative and positive liberty.

In sum, civic republicanism came to be associated with political independence (freedom from domination by larger political societies), active citizenship, a diverse commercial and civic life, a strong sense of patriotism and civic duty or civic virtue, social, and later constitutional, checks and balances, and a diversity of political institutions that represented a fusion of the elements of other types of unitary regime.

Among these themes, the concept of virtue is key. Machiavelli, for example, is notorious for rejecting the Christian morality of the later middle ages and the early modern period, which instructed political leaders about the moral virtues they should exemplify in their conduct and rule. In this so-called 'Mirror for Princes' literature, Christian moralists basically urged political leaders to adhere to the same set of virtues—such as justice, mercy, humility, magnanimity, charity, and forgiveness—that all other Christians of good character were expected to obey. Machiavelli argued that these virtues would be disastrous in practice for a ruler because they would not work in the context of political life, and especially in the anomic context of relationships between principalities or nation states. The result would be to expose one's people to hardship, suffering, and domination; precisely the opposite of the supreme virtue that is expected in a leader, namely the safety and independence of one's people. A new kind of distinctively political virtue was called for, Machiavelli argued, if statecraft were to be both successful and in the service of the common good. Political virtue would displace Christian moral virtue from the public realm and relegate it to private or family life.

Both the distinctiveness and the content of civic virtue has been a topic of ongoing dispute in the republican tradition. Later republican theorists disagreed deeply with Machiavelli's account of what virtues were required of republican citizens, to say nothing of the *Realpolitik* that he embraces in his advice to princes. In his account of civic virtue, Machiavelli places a strong emphasis on virility, manliness, and the bold decisiveness to seize and control fortune or the chance appearance of opportunity amid the normally uncontrollable flow of political events in time. In a quite different republican thinker like Rousseau, by contrast, civic virtue has to do with the self-affirmation that comes from doing one's duty and exemplifying mutuality and solidarity toward one's fellow citizens.

Many contemporary historians of the early modern and renaissance periods, such as Hans Baron, J. G. A. Pocock, and Quentin Skinner, have focused attention on the spread of republican thinking into the seventeenth and eighteenth centuries (Baron 1966; Pocock 1975; Skinner 1978; van Gelderen and Skinner 2002). Civic republicanism became the main ideological foe of monarchy (with its theories of natural law hierarchy and the divine right of kings) in the nation states of northern Europe. It was instrumental in the Puritan revolution in England in the 1640s and again in the Glorious Revolution of 1687. It was even more significant, perhaps, in the French Revolution a century later. Great political theorists such as Harrington, Montesquieu, and Rousseau may be properly seen as civic republicans, as can a host of lesser thinkers during this period (Pocock 1975; Keohane 1980; Ashcraft 1986; Robbins 1959; and Patten 1996).

Both the English and the French deposed and executed a king (Charles I and Louis XVI respectively) and set up a republic. After a taste of radical republicanism (1640−60) and a brief restoration of absolute monarchy (1660−89), the English, in their second revolution of the seventeenth century, did neither; but they did install a new royal family with considerably less power than earlier monarchs, and they shifted toward a much more mixed and parliamentary system than ever before. Republican forms and ideas had clearly taken root, even if the austere vision of the radical protestant reformers had not. A few years later Montesquieu would take England to be a model of an ideally mixed constitutional regime. Republican thinking continued to flourish in the aftermath of the French Revolution and well into the nineteenth century. Both Hegel (in his *Philosophy of Right*) and Tocqueville further refined the theory of complex constitutionalism and can be considered civic republicans, although they have each been assigned to different schools of thought by other commentators.

By the mid-1800s, however, a number of new bodies of social and political theory were edging republicanism aside. These included Bentham's utilitarianism, the writings of the capitalist political economists, modern liberals such as Benjamin Constant, John Stuart Mill, Wilhelm von Humboldt, and in some respects Tocqueville, and of course the rise of socialism and Marxism. Probably the last strong influence of republicanism to be seen in Europe was in the various uprisings of 1848; the conservative reactions to those movements and the development of work that was much better able to address the emerging problems of industrial capitalism put republicanism into decline both as a school of political theory and as a revolutionary movement.[8]

Turning to North America, classical republicanism has been a very important strand in American political thought. For many years mainstream American historians had argued that American political culture had always been dominated by Lockeian liberalism, or proto-liberalism—a social contract theory based on the idea of natural right of the individual to protection of life, liberty, and property. This view found brilliant expression in the 1950s in the work of Louis Hartz (1955; Kramnick 1990). Beginning in the 1970s, however, a number of American historians including Bailyn (1965), Wood (1972), and others took issue with the Hartz thesis and showed that there was as strong a civic republican influence in the political pamphlet literature prior to the revolution and in the thinking of many who wrote and defended the new constitution.[9]

We now know that republican ideas and writings had a significant influence on the American revolutionaries and on the political culture of the colonies more generally in the early and mid-eighteenth century. It not only helped to justify the American revolution, but also had a significant guiding effect on the design of a new form of government, the United States of America. In the debate over the ratification of the new constitution various strands of American republicanism and liberalism came to the fore. Writing to find a consensus, but in defense of ratification, James Madison, Alexander Hamilton, and John Jay in the *Federalist Papers* produced a fascinating amalgam of republican and liberal thinking. Republican ideas and influences can be found not only in writings of the revolutionary and the constitutional periods, but also in American jurisprudence and social reform movements during the first half of the nineteenth century.

In particular, as Michael Sandel has shown, early nineteenth-century American law and economic policy were both animated by the civic republican project of promoting civic life and the flourishing and moral development of individuals through civic life and through the exercise of

---

[8] The economics associated with civic republicanism was distinctly pre-industrial in its emphasis on national economic self-sufficiency and on the virtues of agrarianism over urban industrialism; Gandhi was well aware of republican writings and perhaps is one of the few twentieth century revolutionaries to take them seriously. And perhaps this tradition could have some lessons for a post-industrial world.

[9] For critical perspectives see Pangle (1988) and Diggins (1984).

civic virtue.[10] Certain social and economic practices that were seen as threatening to the virtuous habits, the *moeurs* (morals/manners), of the republic were legally proscribed or regulated for that reason.

This is particularly significant for our purposes because the origins of public health in the United States date from precisely this period. Both the legal foundations and the intellectual leadership of early American public health were fashioned in this civic republican milieu (Gostin 2000b). Just as civic republicanism was gradually supplanted by utilitarianism beginning as early as the 1840s, so too did public health become an increasingly technical, methodologically oriented field. Born out of a republican vision of health and free citizens fit for public life, public health eventually came to be devoted to the moral vision of freeing a population of individuals from the burden of disease in order that they may lead more productive and happier private lives.

It is precisely this historic shift of moral vision that needs revisiting and reconsideration in public health and public health ethics today. It met the needs of its time and arguably put public health into a more realistic posture in the face of the increasing dominance of industrial capitalism. It also rid public health of various religious influences and a tenor of 'moralism' that is elitist and oppressive (Marone 1997). Republicanism, like its contemporary nephew, communitarianism, is prone to such moralism, and that is one of its signal weaknesses that must be kept in check and handled very carefully. However, to borrow a phrase from Robert Putnam (2000: 22–4), I believe that the conceptual framework of civic republicanism can give us access to a 'bridging' as well as to a 'bonding' conception of community and sociality. That is to say, it can be made serviceable in the context of a diverse pluralistic society that morally requires—and pragmatically and political demands—respect for difference and an emphasis on the forms of representational and deliberative policymaking that can encompass that respect even as the policies address common problems.

There are four principal concepts that the tradition of civic republicanism has to offer public health ethics. Two such notions have been identified so far: first, the notion of freedom as life in the absence of arbitrary power and domination; second, the flip side of the concept of domination, the notion of relationships of mutuality and reciprocity wherein individuals can flourish and grow. When Karl Marx described a communal mode of life in which 'the

---

[10] M. Sandel (1984); for critical assessments see Pettit (1998) and Allen and Regan (1998).

free development of each depends upon the free development of all,' he was perhaps speaking less for what Marxism would later become than he was for what republicanism had been.

The primary evil for republicanism is not particular behaviors that violate moral rules, but the deleterious effects of domination and arbitrary power. For republicanism the moral life is a journey toward self-realization and human flourishing in the company of others; it is not the successful passing of each day without transgression. The modern day version of this perspective surely tends in the direction of respecting diversity in a pluralistic society and seeking a framework of values in which each individual can claim equal membership, standing, and respect. It does not tend in the direction of imposing one group's moral or religious code (even in the guise of health) on to other groups, using the authoritative power of the state (even in the guise of the public health apparatus) to do so.

The third republican concept that has a place in public health ethics is the idea of civic virtue. The fourth is the concept of the public. The remainder of this chapter will be devoted to a discussion of these concepts.

It is important to appreciate the interrelationship that civic virtue and the public have. The relationship is, to use an overworked word, dialectical. Civic virtue is a practical form of life that shapes human motivation and self-identity. The practice of civic virtue forges citizens. Citizens are psychological and social embodiments of civic virtue. Citizens, in turn, act in common in such a way as to create the public space. But, and here is the circularity, the public space is necessary for the practice of civic virtue in the first place. Republicanism gives us a vision of a form of political and moral life and political and moral agents that is virtuously circular once it gets going, but it is very difficult to fathom how it could ever get started, or evolve from some non-republican setting. And yet it did historically, and it may again.

3.4. Civic Virtue

Ethical and political theories differ in the use they make of the concept of virtue in at least three ways. First, they differ in exactly what they take the concept of virtue to signify. Second, theories differ in the traits or characteristics that they identify as important virtues. Fully developed theories of virtue often contain elaborate classification schemes to identify different types of virtues across the full range of human life. Different lists of virtues direct conduct toward different patterns of behavior, and they make up different understandings of the nature of the good life. Finally, some virtues are said to be universally applicable to all persons, to human beings as such, while other virtues attach to particular social roles, offices, or functions.

What is a virtue? In some accounts, it is primarily a psychological and a motivational concept. I have a feeling of courage and am thus predisposed to act bravely in the face of danger. I have an inner sense of justice and so I do not treat others unfairly even though it may be in my advantage to do so. The underlying psychological mechanisms at work in the operation of virtue are also multi-faceted. Virtues may be defined as moral beliefs or reflective commitments that a person comes to accept on the basis of deliberation and experience. Or virtues may be said to operate less rationally and deliberately; they may be more like habits or responses to situations not requiring much reflection or weighing of pros and cons, costs and benefits. Virtues on this type of account are usually said to come from a good upbringing and from socialization in a morally wholesome tradition or culture. Some hold that the possession of a virtue is itself sufficient to guarantee ethical conduct in accordance with that virtue; others regard a virtue as a necessary but not a sufficient condition to produce good conduct; additional motivations, inducements, or incentives may be needed too. Brave men may risk their lives in battle, but they also know that they will be punished severely if they desert and are caught.

One particularly illuminating philosophical account of virtue has been developed by Alasdair MacIntyre (1981). He argues that virtues should not be seen as things somehow residing internally in the mind (rational motivation) or in the heart (emotional motivation), but rather as features that accompany our interpretation of the meaning of rule-governed social and cultural 'practices.' A practice is a pattern of conduct that a given cultural tradition identifies with the meeting of human needs and with the pursuit of human excellences. There are trusted, established, and rule-governed ways in which all variety of activities in human life can be performed. These can be learned and they can be done correctly or incorrectly, effectively or ineffectively, well or badly. There are, for example, ways of raising crops, fighting wars, rearing children, organizing groups of persons to accomplish complex tasks, representing clients in court—practices all. Each of these practices is associated with goods that are external to the practice and goods

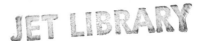

that are internal to it. The practice of medicine has the curing of disease, the restoration of function, and the relief of suffering as goods that are external to it in the sense that medical practice is the means to those ends. But medicine also has goods that are not contingently related to its practice, but are constitutive of it. These goods may be said to be discerning powers of observation, analytic reasoning and diagnostic skills, empathy, discretion, caring, courage, and the ability to be faithful to another in a time of extreme vulnerability and need.

Following MacIntyre, I define a virtue as a human excellence associated with certain social practices and forms of life. I am not interested in inventorying the psychological motivation of the moral person. Virtues are not 'inside' a person's head. They are manifested in the way a person engages in social conduct and the normative or rule-governed practices a person pursues, and the excellence achieved within the conduct of the practice as well as the success achieved as a result of applying its powers.

Similarly, civic virtue is neither a belief nor a feeling, but rather a way of living and being in the political world. It is the excellence pursued in the practice of citizenship, while the good internal to that practice is the common good. Civic virtue is a way of life that sustains the space of the republic, and it is only within the space of the republic that the practice of citizenship and the pursuit of the common good are possible. Civic virtue is the human excellence that makes the republic possible and sustains the common good internal to the practice of citizenship.

Civic virtue must not only be understood and embraced by political elites but also by ordinary citizens, for it is finally their voice and their sense of morality that directs the republic as a whole. A republic without a widespread sense of civic virtue among its citizenry was not viable or sustainable. It would inevitably break down and give way to some other type of regime if it were to succumb to 'corruption,' which in the republican lexicon does not mean merely using office for personal gain, but something much more fundamental—a loss of the capacity to work and sacrifice for the sake of the good of the republic and the good of one's fellow citizens. Corruption is not merely betraying the republic, but losing sight of it, erasing it. This is a profound loss of political imagination. It is also a loss of the capacity to care about the common good.

On the basis of these considerations, I draw the following conclusion. In the republican tradition, and in the political theory that should under gird public health ethics, the common good can be understood as the good that is internal to the practice of citizenship, civic virtue is excellence in the pursuit of that good. Moreover, the practice of citizenship requires the creation of public space, for it is something that individuals can engage in only as members of, and in the context of, a public. These are complex formulations. Let me try to unpack them further.

The activities of citizenship are speaking and listening, deliberating, setting rules of conduct, prioritizing and allocating resources, winning, losing, compromising; in short, Aristotle's 'ruling and being ruled in turn.' Citizenship and the life of civic virtue do *not* have some external state of affairs called the 'common good' as their instrumental objective. The common good is constituted by the proper institutionalization and functioning of citizenship and by the proper embedding of civic virtue in the lifeworld.

The common good is not a notion that sets up a test for particular policies or particular actions to meet (as does the parallel concept of 'the public interest' in utilitarianism or liberal welfarism). It is not an outcome or an effect. However, the notion of the common good does provide a touchstone for judging and appraising a particular policy or decision. It appraises policy against criteria such as non-domination, non-arbitrariness, reasonable authority, mutual respect, reciprocity, and equity.

Contemporary utilitarianism tends to define interests or 'utilities' abstractly across a population of individuals who have, as it were, only external or instrumental relationships to those interests. Utilitarianism also tends to ignore the distributional patterns in which these interests are fulfilled or their impact on discrete individual persons as such; it focuses instead on the net maximization of satisfaction or interest fulfillment in the aggregate. (Robbins 1962; Walsh 1996). By contrast, the judgments that make up republican policy appraisal are judgments of fittingness, character, and appropriateness. They must take into consideration the conditions of power and meaning that constitute the identity and interests of each person as a unique individual. They are at the political boundary between moral and aesthetic judgment. As such, they cannot be the *only* means of policy appraisal, in public health or in any other area. But neither should they be left out altogether (Nussbaum 1995).

3.5. The Concept of the Public

We have inherited a group of concepts from classical Greek and Roman political thought that were developed in order to understanding the human capacity for—and practical experience of—shared forms of life, purposes, and predicaments. Classical political theorists invented these concepts to capture their experience of the public that their own history, institutions, and environment made possible. These concepts (*polis, politeia, polites*, in Greek; *civitas, res publica, cive* in Latin) are the roots of our own terms—political, public, civic, common, community, citizen, and republic. We retain these terms as central to our political vocabulary—in fact they have been largely kept alive by the influence of the civic republican tradition—but their meaning can and has changed (Wolin 1968). Similarly, we still have the cultural and institutional reality of the public within our own political experience; it remains a permanent possibility of the way in which human beings can organize themselves in large numbers, but it certainly is not a necessary feature of human society and in the modern world its existence is fleeting and fugitive at best (Jennings 1981).

Shared purposes or problems are not the same as individual purposes or problems that happen to overlap for large numbers of people. Of course, they do affect persons as individuals and as members of smaller groups, but they also affect the constitution of a 'people,' a population of individuals as a structured social whole. An aggregation of individuals becomes a people, a public, a political community when it is capable of recognizing common purposes and problems in this way; and what allows it to have this kind of political understanding and imagination has largely to do with a dynamic interplay between what I shall call *action* and *structure* over time.

A public has a structure comprised of norms, networks, institutions, and traditions.[11] That structure is durable; it is made up of institutional facts that provide a life–world within which political actors (leaders, representatives, and citizens) can engage in rule-governed practices of precisely the sort that involve virtues. Yet the structure of a public must adapt to a changing natural,

---

[11] Note that it is grammatically necessary, albeit awkward, in English to refer to 'the public' as a noun and not merely an adjective modifying something else; or else one must resort to metaphors such as 'the public space' or 'the public sphere.' This grammatical nominalization is one source of the tendency to reify this concept, a danger to which I will return.

social, and technological environment. It is a kind of dynamic form (like a fountain or waterfall) as distinct from a static form (like a statue). No single individual actor alone can normally change this structure (there are a few notable historical exceptions), but many actors over time can and do transform the public structure of norms, networks, and institutions. Indeed, it is an essential feature of the public as a structure that it be produced and reproduced over time by the praxis of its members or citizens. At the same time, and without contradiction, the public structure comprises a large part of the cultural matrix within which human beings are socialized and educated, and take on their self- and social identity as 'citizens.' The public produces and reproduces citizens even as citizens produce and reproduce the public.

The praxis that has the effect of re-producing and changing the public has two modes. The first is political action itself—collective, cooperative efforts, arrived at through deliberation and the advice of experts. Political action may aim to solve common problems, achieve common purposes or goods, and most fundamentally to change the constitutional structure of the public itself by redistributing power, altering the boundaries of membership, and redistributing emphasis among the multiple values that any public encompasses. An example of this fundamental kind of political action would be a relative shift from an emphasis on individual liberty in public life and public policy to an emphasis on equality. Or, closer to the domain of public health, an example of what I mean here by political action would be a shift from accepting high levels of risk to human health or the environment to tolerating only lower levels of risk in our lives; such a shift is sometimes referred to succinctly as the 'precautionary principle.'

The second, and equally important, mode of praxis whereby actors dynamically change the structure of the public by reproducing it over time is political theorizing or political interpretation. This is the interpretation and reinterpretation of the norms and institutions that do exist and are constitutive of the public structure, as well as an interpretation of the problems, purposes and policies that the public *should* have because they are consistent with its fundamental norms and values. This work of critical interpretation and reinterpretation is essential because the public structure does not exist only in and through the actions that its members take; it also exists in and through the intentions and ideas that its members have about it and about themselves. The public is an 'imagined community' (Anderson 1991); a form of the social imaginary. The public is conceptually dependent upon—'constituted by'—the exercise of the sociological (I would prefer to say, political) imagination.[12]

3.5.1. The Public as Residual to the Private

There are many available ways of defining and understanding the idea of the public; some have developed within the liberal tradition itself as it has come to appreciate the limitations of a purely aggregative notion. We in the field of public health ethics need to begin the work of distinguishing and characterizing these various notions, for they are too often conflated and used interchangeably.

One concept of the public that many thinkers use as a step beyond the merely aggregative notion is the idea of the public as a space of external goods, or externalities. The resources within this domain do not belong to particular individuals, and the attitude that results from this is one of *carte blanche* exploitation (they don't belong to anyone) instead of being one of mutual responsibility (they belong to everyone). The public in this sense is a danger because if the resources contained within it are important (like clean air or water) they are at risk of depletion and degradation. Ever in jeopardy, ever an orphan, the public understood as the space of external goods calls forth collective action, *faute de mieux*, in the wake of market failure and restraint based on self-interest.

Different from external goods or externalities, another conception of the public developed by economists, public choice theorists, and others working out of the liberal welfarist and utilitarian tradition, resides in the concept of 'public goods.' Public goods, like external goods, are not easy or efficient to get private parties to pay for on a commodity basis. They benefit everyone to one degree or another, but no one acting in a private capacity can be said to be responsible for their care and maintenance. So they are vulnerable to over-use and under-support, the so-called 'free rider' problem. National defense, environmental pollution, universal education, natural monopolies

[12] Thus far the scholar in the field of public health who has done the most to revitalize the republican tradition and its sense of the nature of public life and the common good is Dan E. Beauchamp (1976, 1985, and 1988). In his writings, in fact, there seem to be several conceptions of the public, community, and the common good at work, and he does not pay sufficient attention, in my view, to the tasks of conceptual differentiation, definition, and analysis.

caused by technology, such as communication broadcasts, and the like are often categorized as public goods in this sense.

In public health, maintenance of herd immunity by continuing a mandatory vaccination program for children despite the drop off of new cases of infection, would be an example of a public good. Left to itself, the interests and incentives at work in the private health care system might well let herd immunity weaken or disappear, thereby subjecting the population to the risk of epidemic. In advocating to maintain high levels of herd immunity, the public health authority tends to a public good the private sector on its own would not be able to protect.

These various liberal conceptions of the public—as an aggregation of individuals, as the space of externalities and as the public goods that cannot practically or efficiently be bought and sold—provide us with no robust normative position on the intrinsic significance of the public realm.[13] This way of understanding what is public rests, at best, on morally weak considerations of prudence and contingency. They are residual notions, while civic republicanism offers what I would call a transformative conception of the public. Using the well-known thought experiment called the tragedy of the commons (Hardin 1968), I propose to explain that distinction and try to draw out a contrast between these conceptions of the public and a more adequate conception that can be recovered from, and developed out of, the republican tradition.

3.5.2. The Public and the Commons

Imagine a large tract of rich grassland owned by no one and surrounded by several dairy farms. From time immemorial the farmers have allowed their cattle to graze some of the time on the common field. Since the grass there is free, whereas they must pay to maintain the food their cattle eat on their own property, the farmers have an incentive to graze their herd on the common as much as possible. On the other hand, overgrazing will eventually destroy the fertility of the soil and the ecosystem of the common

[13] Later in the chapter, I shall consider one additional non-republican conception of the public, a reified or organic notion, that does offer a robust normative position, indeed all too robust, and that is one of its problems. Liberal notions of the public perform bridging functions, but they build bridges that are too narrow and can't bear much weight. Organic notions of the public perform bonding functions, but they bond all too tightly and with a vengeance.

will collapse, leaving less and less grass for everyone until eventually the land will become barren. So each farmer has at least a long term incentive not to over burden the carrying capacity of the common.

If the motivational and behavioral assumptions of most liberal economic theories are correct, the farmers will inevitably be driven to overgraze the land by short term self-interest and fear of losing competitive advantage. The logic of self-interest and insecurity caused by the lack of a common ruler will doom the common, and hence be an irrational outcome as well as an environmentally harmful one. Of course, it could be that the farmers will be able to exercise self-restraint and will spontaneously refrain from taking advantage of the restraint of the other two. This would be a solution of virtue, not so much civic virtue perhaps, but altruism. Otherwise, between sainthood and disaster, there are three possible solutions.

1. *Create a common power.* One solution to prevent the tragedy of the commons was proposed by Thomas Hobbes and other contractarian thinkers long ago. It is to set up a common authority to make and to enforce common rules. This can be done by conquest of the strongest or by collective agreement through a social contract. In effect, the commons would now become the private property of the sovereign and would be protected as such.

2. *Transform the common into private property.* A second solution would be to somehow internalize the cost to the farmers for the use of the common resource. Make the farmers pay for the grass when their cattle graze there rather than allowing them to exploit this resource for free. Or the commons could be subdivided and turned into the private property of each of the farmers in equal shares. This would save the common but with the consequence that there would be no public thing or nothing in common there at all.

3. *Protect the common (resource) by turning it into a common good.* A third logical solution—the republican and democratic one, it seems to me—is to begin group deliberations to come to some kind of civic consensus on regulations and rules of 'using' the commons without using it up. This would make its preservation and maintenance a matter of accepted duty and shared membership. Here the commons would be recognized for the first time not merely as a free resource but as a truly common or mutual good in our shared way of life; something that will benefit

all the parties best and will be sustainable over time, if and only if none of the parties exploit it unduly or unfairly. Here each farmer, for the first time, takes on a dual identity. One is his private identity as a competitive entrepreneur and follower of short term interests.[14] The other is a civic identity as citizen in the face of this new public thing. As a citizen he has not just private interests, but also public duties; not just the virtues of a successful businessman, but also civic virtues that call for the care and stewardship of the ecological health of the commons.

The third solution clarifies the distinction made above between residual and transformative notions of the public. In this transformation, something that is a raw material or resource for use becomes a value for mutual concern and stewardship. This is a gestalt shift in the way in which social (and natural) reality is perceived. Such shifts are the hallmarks of the public as a space of moral and political transactions in the republican tradition.

How has the liberal tradition viewed these three solutions to what is the quintessential problem of political theory, the problem of collective action? The liberal tradition has rejected Hobbesian absolute sovereignty, but is comfortable with a more limited version of collective authority, restrained by electoral competition among elites and the rule of law. The second solution, privatization of the commons, is the preferred solution of free-market liberalism even today. However, many liberals, and many in public health, will reject the third solution with its politics of imagination that goes beyond fear (the key to the first solution) and gain (the key to the second solution). Some will reject it because they consider it an unrealistic and unworkable approach to the tragedy of the commons. This is an empirical question and the jury of political science is still out on it (Green and Shapiro 1994). But others will reject it for a substantial philosophical reason. They are concerned about the repressive, anti-liberal consequences of any concepts of the public that are culturally powerful and normatively resonant. I see the republican conception of the public as a middle way between a political imagination too thin and one too thick. But this concern is not mistaken and to it we now turn.

---

[14] The first and second solutions, the Hobbesian sovereign and the private property/market price system, do not alter the farmers' private identity as entrepreneurs, they merely change their incentive structures.

3.5.3. A Republican Leviathan?

If the residual conceptions of the public we have just been considering are not satisfactory, neither is another way of talking about the public to which many, including some in public health ethics, fall prey. This is a reified concept of the public; it conceives of the public as if it were a natural thing—an organic whole with its own interests, needs, and being—as opposed to a socially constructed, imaginary life–world. Reification—treating social reality as if it were material or natural reality—leads the theorist to predicate to the entity moral, legal, and other normative properties that are predicated to human persons. The public has rights, interests, obligations. It can be harmed or injured. While it is often legally necessary to reify government or corporate agencies in this fashion, at least they have identifiable structures of authority, accountability, and responsibility. Like human persons, they are tangible actors in the social and natural world; they do things that have consequences.

The concept of the public understood as a socially constructed reality is there to provide the space of meaning to guide and identify actors, not to be an actor itself or to have the predicates of human action (intention, purpose, responsibility, and the like) ascribed to it as such. If the public can be said to act, it is in a very indirect and special way, through the purposes and meaning-making of citizens, not on its own accord.

The principal danger of reification is that it sets up an opposition or conflict between the public and the individuals who comprise it. The interests of the public are set against those of individuals or groups. Unnecessary problems of liberty or justice seem to arise. Enormous confusion can ensue when the public becomes equated with the state, the society, or a public health department. Then it is not a conflict between individuals and a bureaucratic agency. It is public health itself as a villain; public health versus individuals rights, interests, and goods. Political reification (almost always uncalled for) intertwines with legal reification (sometimes useful) to compound this confusion. Corporate or governmental interests take on authority and legitimacy that is ethically and philosophically unwarranted because they appear in the guise of a normative conception of the common good or the public interest. A use of metaphors with a reifying effect takes the place of valid ethical justification and argument.

I do not wish to deny that tensions and conflicts do exist or to say that the rights and interests of individuals are never overridden or compromised in political life generally (even in a republic) or in the practice of public health. But the philosophical move of reification is neither the only nor the best way to acknowledge this tension and to theorize it. As an alternative I would suggest the move of *internalizing this tension and dualism within the political and moral agent himself or herself*. The true tension is not between the reified interests of something called the public and the localized interests of individuals. The tension is within the objective situation and the motivational structure (conscience) of each citizen. We are all torn between our private wills and our civic wills, between our interests as isolated individuals or consumers and our moral interests and commitments as members of a community of shared purpose broader than ourselves. This is the symbiosis of the public and the private. In my view, it should not be eliminated, but lived with and worked through. There will always be free riders. And there will also be fanatics of civic virtue. Most of us will be caught in the middle, neither wishing to live in a society of total privatization and selfishness, such as the Ik culture described by Turnbull (1972), nor in a society of total commitment, such as Oceania in Orwell's *Nineteen Eighty-Four*.

3.6. Health and the Common Good

Earlier I maintained that it is only within the space of the republic that the practice of citizenship and the pursuit of the common good are possible. This is a complex and no doubt controversial claim, and it requires further explication. To say that it is only within the space of the republic that the practice of citizenship is possible may be understandable enough. Drawing on no less an authority than Aristotle, the civic republicans were wont to observe that only a politically free people could be citizens and the *polis* or the *res publica* were by definition the only political regimes where the people were free. In monarchies, or in the despotisms of the ancient Persian, Syrian, or Egyptian empires, individuals were 'subjects' not citizens.

But why say that only in a republic is the pursuit of the common good possible? Surely in monarchies there is such a thing as the common good also; some state of affairs that is better for people than other possible states of affairs. But if it makes sense to say that there is no real civic life in a monarchy, that there is no practice of citizenship possible because the constitutive social rules and meanings necessary for citizenship are missing, then all persons in a monarchy are private persons, all lives are private lives, and all goods to be pursued are private goods. National security? A private good of each of us taken seriatim. Literacy and education for all? A private good for each of us, but not a common good for all of us.

And what about health? As Norman Daniels—writing then from a liberal contractarian point of view—has said, health is a primary good in that it allows each individual to attain normal species functioning, and that, in turn, is the key to each individual's capacity to take advantage of the equality of opportunity that a liberal society grants each person as a matter of right (Daniels 1985; see also. Daniels et al. 1999). (In liberal theory, citizens are bearers of rights, not agents engaged in the defining political practice.) Is health a good we have in common, or is it a prerequisite for the individual enjoyment, more accurately, the consumption of various opportunities open to us? Again, the latter formulation would seem to be the appropriate answer so long as we are living in a form of society that does not truly grasp the notion of the public or the common, but only understands a collectivity or an aggregation of private interests. Outside the space of political and moral practices that the tradition has called a republic, there can be no genuinely public health; there can only be a body of expertise employed in the service of increasing the private health states of individuals. Only a republic is socially constructed around the shared perception that there is a common good or a 'public thing' among us to be sustained, nurtured, defended at times, and gradually improved. And the very notion of public health, I suggest, is contained in that form of social imaginary, that form of socially constructed perception and practice.

Of course, when we use the term public health or talk about 'improving public health,' part of what we mean is 'improving the aggregate health status of individuals.' But this is not all that we mean. Because this abstracts away from one of the core defining characteristics that have given the field of public health its distinctive identity historically. When public health talks about health it means a state of biological, psychological, and social functioning of a human organism/person in a social context. The persons whom public health studies and works with are physically embodied and socially embedded entities. The fact that they live in a symbolically constructed space that permits them to imagine a common good and a public health, and hence to orient themselves toward them, is a significant fact for the field of public health to understand as a part of the social embeddedness of the person. The fact that they do not live in such a space is also a fact germane to their health contextually and socially understood.

Therefore the concept of the common good and the notion of the public are essential to the field of public health in two ways. They are necessary components of the field's assessment of the health status and prospects of real people leading messy, encumbered, communally thick or thin lives. Without these notions public health professionals would not know a republic if they saw one. But by the same token, they would not know a despotism or a totalitarian regime either.

The concept of the common good is essential to public health in a second way as well. Without it, public health will not be able to talk seriously about its own professional identity and values. The field of public health relies on the capacity for people in the population to comprehend the meaning of a common danger or a common good. If the people with whom public health has to deal, in whatever society around the world, have lost the capacity to comprehend these ideas, then it will not be possible to either coerce or empower them to undertake the kind of collective institutional and behavioral change that health deficits in the world today manifestly require, from coping with HIV/AIDS to coping with the need to build a long-term care system in the aging societies.

Arguments to justify coercive state authority and arguments to justify legitimate community based initiatives for reducing health risks and health promotion will not be successful if they rely on abstract and universal propositions about rights, obligations, and interests alone. Such arguments will need to appeal more concretely and specifically to ideals and feelings engendered by people's lived experience in various social practices. To the extent that this lived experience is one of privatization and a suspicious, competitive egoism and cynicism, then I submit that public health efforts will have little uptake if they are educational and voluntary, and will prove far too costly and repressive if they involve coercive state action. On the other hand, to the extent that this lived experience is one approaching citizenship and a civic orientation, then such public health efforts will be able to draw upon the civic virtue latent in the population and educational efforts will gain a more positive response, while official public policy will be met with more self-directed or spontaneous obedience and compliance.

If the foregoing analysis is correct, it suggests an interesting notion. Not all societies in the world today closely resemble a republic (although many continue to use that term to name themselves). In fact, very few do. But in any society, no matter what its constitutional form or its political shape, when public health works effectively it must create a small republic within a wider non-republican society and political culture. It must build a bubble of civic virtue and a small space for the political imagination and the common good. These spaces may be transient and fleeting. But wherever public health educators or policy analysts do their work and practice their interventions, there is always the potentiality for the creation of a space for health citizenship.

Public health does not always take advantage of this potentiality, or succeed in actualizing it. At times the effect of public health programs, unfortunately, is to reinforce privatization, competition, and particularistic self-interest. But as an ethical aspiration and guiding ideal, public health should always seek to realize the civic and, so to speak, republican potential that it finds in the polities and civil societies in which it works.

4

Health of the People: The Highest Law?[1]

Lawrence O. Gostin and Lesley Stone

> From my perspective, as a White House official watching the budgetary process, and subsequently as head first of a health care financing agency and then of a public health agency, I was continually amazed to watch as billions of dollars were allocated to financing medical care with little discussion, whereas endless arguments ensued over a few millions for community prevention programs. The sums that were the basis for prolonged, and often futile, budget fights in public health were treated as rounding errors in the Medicare budget.
>
> (William Roper 1994)

Law and ethics in population health are having a renaissance (Gostin 2000a; Reynolds 2003). Once fashionable during the Industrial (Shattuck 1850; Chadwick 1965) and Progressive (Duffy 1990) eras, the ideals of population health began to wither with the rise of liberalism in the late twentieth century (Hamlin 2002). In its place came a sharpened focus on personal and

[1] This chapter is based on the Guest Keynote Address presented by Professor Gostin at the Conference, Health of the People: The Highest Law? 8 January 2004, Queen Elizabeth II Conference Centre, London, England, sponsored by the Nuffield Trust, the UK Public Health Association, and the Faculty of Public Health of the Royal College of Physicians. A briefer version of this chapter appears in Gostin (2004a). For an expanded version of these ideas, see Gostin (2000b, 2002a).

economic freedom. Political attention shifted from population health to individual health and from public health to private medicine.

Signs of revitalization of the field of public health law and ethics can be seen in diverse national and global contexts (Holland and Stewart 1997). International agencies, national governments, and philanthropic organizations are creating centres of excellence in public health law and ethics;[2] initiating broad reforms of antiquated public health laws (WHO 1983; Reynolds 1995; Bidmeade and Reynolds 1997; Monaghan et al. 2003); and calling for effective public health governance systems at the global level (Fidler 1999; Owen 2002; Beaglehole 2003).

The resurgence of interest in population-based law and ethics deserves vigorous attention in modern political and social circles. To facilitate such consideration, it is important to define the field of public health law and ethics and offer a theoretical basis for its practice. Scholars should focus their attention on determining *what* is public health law and ethics and its doctrinal boundaries. This chapter begins the discussion by suggesting a definition for public health law and analysing its components.

Having conceptualized the field, proponents of public health law must develop a well-articulated vision. *Why* should health be a salient public value? This chapter brings focus to this issue, presenting reasons why national and international agencies should create the conditions for a healthy population.

Finally, having discussed what public health law means and why it is important, this chapter outlines the ways in which law can be used to promote the public's health. Given that public health should be an important societal goal, the next question is *how* law can be effective in reducing morbidity and premature mortality. As discussed below, there are at least seven legal tools that can be utilized to promote the public's health. This chapter begins an exploration of the role of public health law in society, which can be fully developed only through the thinking and practice of dedicated public health scholars and advocates.

---

[2] Center for Law and the Public's Health at Georgetown and Johns Hopkins Universities (www.publichealthlaw.net); Centre for Public Health Law at LaTrobe University (http://www.latrobe.edu.au/publichealth/centre_phl/).

4.1. The Problem of Public Health: From Personal Rights to Societal Obligations

> Measures to improve public health, relating as they do to such obvious and mundane matters as housing, smoking, and food, may lack the glamour of high-technology medicine, but what they lack in excitement they gain in their potential impact on health, precisely because they deal with the major causes of common disease and disabilities.
>
> (Geoffrey Rose 1992)

The late twentieth century saw a decline in interest in public health law and ethics. The modern prominence of the libertarian ethic has meant that individual rights are often preferred over common goods. Going forward, population-based health can become revitalized only if we begin to appreciate the reasons why it lost traction in the political sphere.

Public health is a tough sell in the marketplace of ideas (Rose 1985; Burris 1997). There are at least four reasons why politicians and the public under-appreciate public health activities. First, there is *the rescue imperative*. Society is willing to spend inordinately to save the life of a person with a name, face, and history, but less so to save 'statistical lives' (Heinzerling 1998). Medicine seeks to relieve the suffering of particular individuals with life-stories, families, and friends. Public health, on the other hand, often operates at the preventative stage. While it ultimately may save many more lives (e.g., through vaccination programmes), none of those lives is personally identifiable. Second, there is *the technological imperative*—public health services are less appealing than the high technology solutions of microbiology and genetics. For better or worse, many public health measures (including, for example, educational campaigns to encourage healthy behaviours and disease surveillance) do not rely on cutting-edge technology. These measures, therefore, are less likely to capture the attention and imagination of the media and public. The third reason public health is under-appreciated is *the invisibility of public health*. When public health is working well (e.g., safe food, water, and products), its importance tends to be taken for granted. Public health agencies often act in quiet, undramatic ways to assure the conditions for healthy people. Their activities, therefore, are seldom noticed until a crisis emerges. Finally, closely related to the prominence of liberalism, is *the culture of individualism*. Society often values personal goods (individual responsibility, choice, and satisfaction) over public goods (population health and safety). The public health enterprise is unlikely to gain political support when the prevailing ideology prefers individual freedom, less government, and less taxation. These factors make generating political activity and popular interest in public health issues difficult.

The flourishing of libertarian thought during the late twentieth century warrants closer attention. This was a time when scholars had great influence in shaping ideas about the primacy of the individual. Both ends of the political spectrum celebrated the values of free will and personal choice. The political left espoused the virtues of civil liberties, stressing autonomy, privacy, and liberty. At the same time, the political right espoused the virtues of economic liberty, stressing freedom of contract, property privileges, and competitive markets. Personal interests in self-determination attained the status of 'rights'. In this intellectual environment, the individual's own interests often prevailed over the interests of family, community, or country.

Certainly, the power and importance of individual freedom is beyond dispute. However, insufficient attention has been given to the equally strong values of partnership, citizenship, and community. We need to recapture a classic republican tradition that emphasizes communal obligations in addition to self-interest. As members of a society we all have a common bond. Our responsibility is not simply to defend our own right to be free from economic and personal restraint. We also have an obligation to protect and defend the community against threats to health, safety, and security. Each member of society owes a duty—one to another—to promote the common good. And each member benefits from participating in a well-regulated society that reduces risks that all members share. The protection and satisfaction gained from living in a community where public health is recognized as an important value should outweigh the individual self-interest in looking out only for oneself.

4.2. Public Health and the Law: A Theory and a Definition

Liberty does not import an absolute right in each person to be, at all times and in all circumstances, wholly freed from restraint. There are manifold restraints to which every person is necessarily subject for the common good. On any other basis organized society could not exist with safety to its members . . . A fundamental principle of the social compact is that the whole people covenants with each citizen, and each citizen with the whole people, that all shall be governed by certain laws for the common good, and that government is instituted for the common good, for the protection, safety, prosperity and happiness of the people, and not for the profit, honor or private interests of any one man, family or class of men.

(Justice John Harlan 1905)

To overcome the general population's lethargy regarding public health and make a strong argument for shifting the balance away from the individual and toward the common good requires a robust understanding of public health. In defining the relevant terms (public health law, public health, and the common good), we begin to structure the debate. Public health law has been defined as follows:

The legal powers and duties of the state to create the conditions for people to be healthy (e.g., to identify, prevent, and ameliorate significant risks to health in the population) and the limitations on the power of the state to constrain the autonomy, privacy, liberty, proprietary, or other legally protected interests of individuals for the protection or promotion of community health.

(Gostin 2000b)

Through this definition, we suggest five essential characteristics of public health law:

1. *Government*—Public health is a special responsibility of government, in collaboration with partners in the community, business, the media, and academia (Institute of Medicine 2003).
2. *Populations*—Public health focuses on the health of populations rather than individual patients.
3. *Services*—Public health deals with the provision of population-based services grounded on the scientific methodologies of public health (e.g., biostatistics and epidemiology).
4. *Power*—Public health authorities possess the power to regulate individuals and businesses for the protection of the community.

5. *Limitations*—The power of public health authorities to regulate is not absolute, but bounded by legally protected individual interests.

A systematic understanding of public health law requires an examination of the terms 'public health' and the 'common good'. The word 'public' in public health has two overlapping meanings—one that explains the entity that takes primary responsibility for the public's health, and another that explains who has a legitimate expectation to receive the benefits. The government has primary responsibility for the public's health. The government is a 'public' entity that acts on behalf of the people and gains its legitimacy through a political process. A characteristic form of 'public' or state action occurs when a democratically elected government exercises powers or duties to protect or promote the population's health.

The population as a whole has a legitimate expectation to benefit from public health services. The population is served by the government and holds the state accountable for a meaningful level of health protection. Once brought to the electorate's attention, public health should possess broad appeal because it is truly a universal aspiration. In particular cases, however, what best serves the population may not always be in the individual interest of each of its members. And it is for this reason that public health is highly political. What constitutes 'enough' health? What kinds of services? How will services be paid for and distributed? What risks are significant enough to warrant governmental intervention? These remain political questions that confront each government as it sets public health policy.

If individual interests are to give way to communal interests in healthy populations, it is important to understand the value of 'the common' and 'the good'.

The field of public health would profit from a vibrant conception of 'the common' that sees public interests as more than the aggregation of individual interests. A nonaggregative understanding of public goods recognizes that everyone has a stake in living in a society that regulates risks that all share.

As members of society, we have common goals that go beyond our narrow interests. Individuals have a stake in healthy and secure communities where they can live in peace and well-being. An unhealthy or insecure community may produce harms that affect all, such as increased crime and violence, impaired social relationships, and a less productive workforce. Consequently, people may have to forgo a little bit of self-interest in exchange for the protection and satisfaction gained from sustaining healthier and safer communities.

The most famous tale of the disaster that awaits a society wherein each pursues his or her own unfettered interest is Hardin's Tragedy of the Commons (Hardin 1968). Where a resource is finite (a commons upon which to graze cattle), it is in each person's individual interest to use the resource maximally (graze as many cattle as one can buy). Yet in doing so, the resource will be depleted (overgrazing will lead to a barren field) and all will starve. Similarly, in the context of health, industries have few economic incentives to protect the environment because clean-air measures are usually costly. Yet the public interest is better served by restricting pollution. Likewise, an individual may have an interest in refusing a vaccination and avoiding the slight risk of adverse effects. If most of his or her neighbours agree to be vaccinated, the individual gains from 'herd-immunity'. A tragedy of the commons emerges when enough individuals refuse vaccination so that herd immunity is lost. Thus, individual indulgence in 'freedoms' can harm not only the risk-taker, but the larger community.

We also need to better understand the concept of 'the good' sought through public health. In medicine, the meaning of 'the good' is defined purely in terms of the individual's wants and needs. It is the patient, not the physician or family, who decides the appropriate course of action. In public health, the meaning of 'the good' is far less clear. Who gets to decide in a given case which value is more important—freedom or health? One strategy for public health decision-making would be to allow each person to decide, but this would thwart many public health initiatives. For example, if individuals could decide whether to permit reporting of personal information to the health department, many may choose to opt out, resulting in inadequate disease surveillance.

One way forward is to promote greater community involvement in public health decision-making, so that policy formation becomes a genuinely civic endeavour (Callahan and Jennings 2002). Citizens would make the choices necessary to safeguard their communities through civic participation, open fora, and capacity-building to solve local problems. Public involvement should result in stronger support for health policies and encourage citizens to take a more active role in protecting themselves and the health of their neighbours.

Public health, therefore, places special responsibility on government to serve the health needs of populations, as discussed below. It is highly political, so that public health advocates should not shy from energetic, ongoing involvement in the political process. It is also highly participatory, in order that advocates should closely collaborate with affected communities.

4.3. Public Health's Vision: Why Population Health should be a Salient Public Value

> The success or failure of any government in the final analysis must be measured by the well-being of its citizens. Nothing can be more important to a state than its public health; the state's paramount concern should be the health of its people.
>
> (Franklin Delano Roosevelt 1932, in Tobey 1939)

The public health community takes it as an act of faith that health must be society's overarching value. Yet politicians do not always see it that way, expressing preferences, say, for highways, economic development, and military prowess. The lack of political commitment to population health can be seen in the relatively low public health expenditures in many national budgets (Musgrove et al. 2001). Public health professionals often distrust and shun politicians rather than engage them in discussion about the importance of population health. What is needed is a clear vision of, and rationale for, healthy populations as a political priority.

Why should health be a salient public value, as opposed to other communal goods such as transportation, economic development, or national security? Two interrelated theories support the role of health as a primary value:

1. *A theory of human functioning*—health is a foundation for personal well-being and the exercise of social and political rights; and
2. *A theory of government*—governments are formed primarily to achieve health, safety, and welfare of the population.

4.3.1. Health is Foundational: A Theory of Human Functioning

Health is foundationally important because of its intrinsic value and its singular contribution to the functioning of individuals and the community as a whole (Daniels 1985; Brock and Daniels 1994). Every person understands, at least intuitively, why health is vital to well-being. Health is necessary for much of the joy, creativity, and productivity that a person derives from life. If individuals have physical and mental health they are better able to recreate, socialize, work, and engage in the activities of family and social life that bring meaning and happiness. Certainly, persons with ill-health or disability can lead deeply fulfilling lives, but personal health does facilitate many of life's joys and accomplishments. Every person desires the best physical and mental health achievable, even in the face of existing disease, injury, or disability. The people's health is so basic that human rights norms embrace a right to health (CESCR 2000).

Perhaps not as obviously, however, health is also essential for the functioning of populations. Without minimum levels of health, people cannot fully engage in social interactions, participate in the political process, exercise rights of citizenship, generate wealth, create art, and provide for the common security. A safe and healthy population builds strong roots for a country—its governmental structures, social organizations, cultural endowment, economic prosperity, and national defence. Population health, then, becomes a transcendent value because a certain level of human functioning is a prerequisite for engaging in activities that are critical to the public welfare—social, political, and economic.

Health has an intrinsic and instrumental value for individuals, communities, and entire nations. People aspire to achieve health because of its importance to a satisfying life; communities promote the health of their neighbours for the mutual benefits of social interactions; and nations build health care and public health infrastructures to cultivate a decent and prosperous civilization.

4.3.2. Government's Obligation to Promote Health

Why is it that government has an enduring obligation to protect and promote the public's health? People form governments for their common defence, security, and welfare—goods that can only be achieved through collective action. Public health is a classic case of a general communal provision because public funds are expended to benefit all or most of the population without any specific distribution to individuals (Walzer 1983).

A political community stresses a shared bond among members: organized society safeguards the common goods of health, welfare, and security, while members subordinate themselves to the welfare of the community as a whole (Beauchamp 1988). Public health can be achieved only through collective action, not through individual endeavour. Acting alone, individuals cannot assure even basic levels of health. Any person of means can procure many of the necessities of life—for example, food, housing, clothing, and even medical care. Yet no single individual can assure his or her health. Meaningful protection and assurance of the population's health require communal effort. The community as a whole has a stake in environmental protection, hygiene and sanitation, clean air and surface water, uncontaminated food and drinking water, safe roads and products, and control of infectious disease. These collective goods, and many more, are essential conditions for health. Yet these benefits can be secured only through organized action on behalf of the people.

Therefore, political officials are at least putatively committed to securing health for the population, and members of the community are committed to bear the necessary burdens. The collective efforts of the body politic to protect and promote the population's health represent a central theoretical tenet of what we call public health ethics.

4.4. Law as a Tool to Protect the Public's Health: Models of Public Health Intervention

> At the heart of the well-regulated society was a plethora of bylaws, ordinances, statutes, and common law restrictions regulating nearly every aspect of economy and society . . . [Regulations in a good society] granted to public officials the power to guarantee public health (securing the population's well-being, longevity, and productivity). Public health regulation . . . was the central component of a reigning theory and practice of governance committed to the pursuit of the people's welfare and happiness in a well-ordered society and polity.
>
> (William J. Novak 1996)

Given that government has an obligation to provide the conditions for people to be healthy, what tools are at its disposal? There are at least seven models for legal intervention designed to prevent injury and disease, encourage healthful behaviours, and generally promote the public's health. Although legal interventions can be effective, they often raise critical social, ethical, or constitutional concerns that warrant careful study. Each model varies in terms of its coerciveness. Providing information to the public, for example, is less intrusive than placing a tax on disfavoured activities. Still more coercive is direct regulation forbidding or requiring certain actions subject to the full weight of the state. Depending on the severity of the public health problem at which the intervention is aimed, proportional levels of state action may be appropriate and politically acceptable. Public health law is intellectually enticing precisely because it is so difficult, involving complex tradeoffs between individual and collective interests.

4.4.1. Model 1: The Power to Tax and Spend

The power to tax and spend is ubiquitous in national constitutions, providing government with an important regulatory technique. The power to spend supports the public health infrastructure consisting of a well-trained work-force, electronic information and communications systems, rapid disease surveillance, laboratory capacity, and response capability (CDC 2002a). The state can also set health-related conditions for the receipt of public funds. For example, government can grant funds for highway construction or other public works projects on the condition that the recipients meet designated safety requirements.[3]

The power to tax provides inducements to engage in beneficial behaviour and disincentives to engage in risky activities. Tax relief can be offered for health-producing activities such as medical services, childcare, and charitable contributions. At the same time, tax burdens can be placed on the sale of hazardous products such as cigarettes, alcoholic beverages, and firearms. Studies demonstrate that taxation policy has a significant influence on healthful or risk behaviours, particularly among young people (Fox and Schaffer 1991).

Despite their undoubted effectiveness, the spending and taxing powers are not entirely benign. Taxing and spending can be seen as coercive because

---

[3] *South Dakota v. Dole*, 483 U.S. 203 (1987).

the government wields significant economic power. They can also be viewed as inequitable if rich people benefit while the poor are disadvantaged. Some taxing policies serve the rich, the politically connected, or those with special interests (e.g., tax preferences for energy companies or tobacco farmers). Other taxes penalize the poor because they are highly regressive. For example, almost all public health advocates support cigarette taxes, but the people who shoulder the principal financial burden are disproportionately indigent and are often in minority groups.

4.4.2. Model 2: The Power to Alter the Informational Environment

The public is bombarded with information that influences life's choices, and this undoubtedly affects health and behaviour (Institute of Medicine 2001). The government has several tools at its disposal to alter the informational environment, encouraging people to make more healthful choices about diet, exercise, cigarette smoking, and other behaviours.

First, government, as a health educator, uses communication campaigns as a major public health promotion strategy. Health education campaigns, like other forms of advertising, are persuasive communications; instead of promoting a product or a political philosophy, public health campaigns promote safer, more healthful behaviours. Prominent campaigns include safe driving, safe sex, and nutritious diets.

Second, government can require businesses to label their products to include: instructions for safe use, disclosure of contents or ingredients, and health warnings. For example, government requires businesses to explain the dosage and adverse effects of pharmaceuticals, reveal the nutritional and fat content of foods, and warn consumers of the health risks of smoking and drinking alcoholic beverages.

Finally, government can limit harmful or misleading information in private advertising. The state can ban or regulate advertising of potentially harmful products such as cigarettes, firearms, and even high-fat foods. Advertisements can be deceptive or misleading by, for example, associating dangerous activities such as smoking with sexual, adventurous, or active images. Advertisements can also exacerbate health disparities by, for example, targeting product messages to vulnerable populations such as children, women, or minorities.

To many public health advocates, there is nothing inherently wrong with or controversial in ensuring that consumers receive full and truthful information. Yet not everyone believes that public funds should be expended, or the veneer of government legitimacy used, to prescribe particular social orthodoxies—sex, abortion, smoking, high-fat diet, or sedentary lifestyle. (This sentence makes it seem like public funds are prescribing sex, abortion, smoking, etc., rather than safe sex, no smoking, low-fat diet, etc. I don't think it makes sense to call 'sex, abortion, smoking' etc., 'social orthodoxies'). Labelling requirements seem unobjectionable, but businesses strongly protest compelled disclosure of certain kinds of information. For example, should businesses be required to label foods as genetically modified? Genetically modified foods have not been shown to be dangerous to humans, but the public demands a 'right to know'. Advertising regulations restrict commercial speech, thus implicating businesses' right to 'freedom of expression'. The US Supreme Court, for example, has strongly supported the 'right' to convey 'truthful' commercial information.[4] Courts in most liberal democracies, however, do not afford protection to corporate speech.[5] There is, after all, a distinction between political and social speech (which deserve rigorous legal protection) and commercial speech. The former is necessary for a vibrant democracy, while the latter is purchased and seeks primarily to sell products for a profit.

4.4.3. Model 3: The Power to Alter the Built Environment

The design of the built or physical environment can hold great potential for addressing the major health threats facing the global community. Public health has a long history in designing the built environment to reduce injury (e.g., workplace safety, traffic calming, and fire codes), infectious diseases (e.g., sanitation, zoning, and housing codes), and environmentally associated harms (e.g., lead paint and toxic emissions).

Many developed countries are now facing an epidemiological transition from infectious to chronic diseases such as cardiovascular disease, cancer, diabetes, asthma, and depression. The challenge is to shift to communities

---

[4] *Liquormart, Inc. v. Rhode Island*, 517 U.S. 484 (1996).

[5] *Canada Post Corp. v. Epost Innovations Inc.*, 87 C.R.R. (2d) 345 (2001).

designed to facilitate physical and mental well-being. Although research is limited (Srinivasan et al. 2003), we know that environments can be designed to promote liveable cities and facilitate health-affirming behaviour by, for example: encouraging more active lifestyles (walking, biking, and playing); improving nutrition (fruits, vegetables, and avoidance of high-fat, high-calorie foods); decreasing use of harmful products (cigarettes and alcoholic beverages); reducing violence (domestic abuse, street crime, and firearm use); and increasing social interactions (helping neighbours and building social capital) (Ewing et al. 2003).

Critics offer a stinging assessment of public health efforts to alter the built environment: 'The anti-sprawl campaign is about telling [people] how they should live and work, about sacrificing individuals' values to the values of their politically powerful betters. It is coercive, moralistic, nostalgic, [and lacks honesty]' (Postrel 1999). This critique fails to take account of history, norms, and evidence (Perdue et al. 2003). Historically, government has been actively involved in land use planning (Perdue et al. 2004). It is not a matter of whether the state should plan cities and towns, but how. Government makes land use planning decisions to achieve many public purposes, and a nation's health and safety are normatively quite important. The evidence demonstrates that organized societies have a remarkable capacity to plan, shape the future, and help populations increase health and well-being (Jackson 2003). History, theory and empirical evidence do not make it inevitable that the state will, or always should, prefer health-enhancing policies. However, government does have an obligation to carefully consider the population's health in its land use policies.

4.4.4. Model 4: The Power to Alter the Socio-Economic Environment

A strong and consistent finding of epidemiological research is that socio-economic status (SES) is correlated with morbidity, mortality, and functioning (Rogot et al. 1992). SES is a complex phenomenon based on income, education, and occupation. The relationship between SES and health often is referred to as a 'gradient' because of the graded and continuous nature of the association; health differences are observed well into the middle ranges of SES. These empirical findings have persisted across time (Kitagawa and Hauser 1973) and cultures (Marmot et al. 1991), and remain viable today.

For example, researchers have demonstrated socio-economic differentials in the health-related quality of life of Australian children (Spurrier et al. 2003), and similar disparities can be found in vulnerable populations in North America (Department of Health and Human Services 2000) and Europe (Acheson 1998).

Some researchers go further, suggesting the overall level of socio-economic inequality in a society affects health (Wilkinson 1996). That is, societies with fewer inequalities between the rich and poor tend to have superior health status. This phenomenon is apparent in comparisons of health indicators in Organisation for Economic Co-operation and Development (OECD) countries, where life expectancy is higher in countries with well-developed social welfare systems that assure greater equity in resource allocation (Mathers et al. 2003). The explanatory variables are hypothesized to be the lack of social support and cohesion in unequal societies. Although these findings have been challenged empirically (Lynch et al. 2004), some ethicists claim that 'Social justice is good for our health' (Daniels et al. 2000a; Beauchamp 1976).

Despite the strength of evidence, critics express strong objections to policies directed to reducing socio-economic disparities (Deaton 2002). First, they dispute the causal relationship between low SES and poor health outcomes. The poor, they suggest, may have worse health not because of income but for some other reason such as genetic differences, risk behaviours, or reduced access to health care or education. Or, they suggest the causal relationship may be in the other direction—poor health causes low income due to an inability to work or high medical costs. Second, critics infer that reduction in disparities entails redistribution of wealth; greater SES equality necessarily requires programs designed to lift people out of poverty and impoverished conditions. Income reallocation and disruption of competitive markets, they claim, would have adverse economic effects including reduced efficiency and productivity; these economic effects, in turn, could be detrimental to health (Garber 1989; Mellor and Milyo 2002). Consequently, reduction of SES disparities should be a political, not a public health, decision.

Although SES disparities are political questions, the evidence should guide elected officials. Admittedly, the explanatory variables for the relationship between SES and health are not entirely understood. However, waiting for researchers to definitively find the causal pathways would be difficult and time consuming given the multiple confounding factors. This would indefinitely delay policies that could powerfully affect people's health and longevity. What we do know is that the gradient probably involves multiple pathways, each of which can be addressed through social policy (Adler and Newman 2002; Wong et al. 2002). People of low SES experience material disadvantage (e.g., lack of access to food, shelter, and health care); toxic physical environments (e.g., poor conditions at home, work, and in the community); psychosocial stressors (e.g., financial or occupational insecurity and lack of control); and social contexts that influence risk behaviours (e.g., smoking, physical inactivity, high-fat diet, and excessive alcohol consumption). Society can work to try to alleviate each of these determinants of morbidity and premature mortality.

4.4.5. Model 5: Direct Regulation of Persons, Professionals, and Businesses

Government has the power to directly regulate individuals, professionals, and businesses. In a well-regulated society, public health authorities set clear, enforceable rules to protect the health and safety of workers, consumers, and the population at large. Regulation of individual behaviour (e.g., use of seatbelts and motorcycle helmets) reduces injuries and deaths. Licences and permits enable government to monitor and control the standards and practices of professionals and institutions (e.g., doctors, hospitals, and nursing homes). Finally, inspection and regulation of businesses help to assure humane conditions of work, reduction in toxic emissions, and safer consumer products.

Despite its undoubted value, public health regulation of commercial activity is highly contested terrain. Influential economic theories (e.g., laissez-faire and, more recently, a market economy) favour open competition and the undeterred entrepreneur (Epstein 2003). Libertarians view commercial regulation as detrimental to economic growth and social progress. Commercial regulation, they argue, should redress market failures (e.g., monopolistic and other anticompetitive practices) rather than restrain free trade. Yet, public health advocates are opposed to unfettered private enterprise and suspicious of free-market solutions to complex social problems (Gostin and Bloche 2003; Bayer et al. 1995). Unbridled commercialism can produce unsafe work environments; noxious by-products such as waste or pollution; and public nuisances such as unsafe buildings or accumulations of garbage. Regulation is needed to curb the excesses of unrestrained capitalism to ensure reasonably safe and healthful business practices.

4.4.6. Model 6: Indirect Regulation through the Tort System

Attorneys general, public health authorities, and private citizens possess a powerful means of indirect regulation through the tort system. Civil litigation can redress many different kinds of public health harms: environmental damage (e.g., air pollution or groundwater contamination); exposure to toxic substances (e.g. pesticides, radiation, or chemicals); hazardous products (e.g., tobacco or firearms); and defective consumer products (e.g., children's toys, recreational equipment, or household goods). For example, tobacco companies, in 1998, negotiated a Master Settlement Agreement with American states that required massive compensation, with payments totalling US$206 billion through the year 2025 (National Association of Attorneys General 1998).

The goals of tort law, although imperfectly achieved, are frequently consistent with public health objectives. The tort system aims to hold individuals and businesses accountable for their dangerous activities, compensate persons who are harmed, deter unreasonably hazardous conduct, and encourage innovation in product design. Civil litigation, therefore, can provide potent incentives for people and manufacturers to engage in safer, more socially conscious behaviour.

While tort law can be an effective method of advancing the public's health, like any form of regulation, it is not an unmitigated good. First, the tort system imposes economic costs and personal burdens on individuals and businesses (liability and 'transaction' expenses such as court costs and attorneys' fees). Tort costs are absorbed by the enterprise, which often passes the costs onto employees and consumers. Second, tort costs may be so high that businesses do not enter the market, leave the market, or curtail research and development. Society may not be any poorer if tort costs drove out unhealthy enterprises (such as tobacco), but not socially advantageous enterprises (e.g., vaccines and pharmaceuticals). Third, the tort system may be unfair, distributing windfalls to isolated plaintiffs and their attorneys, while failing to compensate the majority of injured people in the population. Studies of the medical malpractice system, for example, demonstrate that large awards are sometimes given to undeserving plaintiffs, while most patients who suffer from medical error are never compensated (Kohn et al. 2000; Weiler et al. 2000).

4.4.7. Model 7: Deregulation: Law as a Barrier to Health

Sometimes laws are harmful to the public's health and stand as an obstacle to effective action. In such cases, the best remedy is deregulation. Politicians may urge superficially popular policies that have unintended health consequences. Consider laws that penalize exchanges or pharmacy sales of syringes and needles. Restricting access to sterile drug injection equipment can fuel the transmission of HIV infection. Similarly, the closure of bathhouses can drive the epidemic underground, making it more difficult to reach gay men with condoms and safe sex literature. Finally, laws that criminalize sex unless the person discloses his or her HIV-status make common sexual behaviour unlawful. The criminal law provides a disincentive for seeking testing and medical treatment, ultimately harming the public's health (Gostin 2004b).

Deregulation can be controversial, since it often involves a direct conflict between public health and other social values such as crime prevention or morality. Drug laws, the closure of bathhouses, and HIV-specific criminal penalties represent society's disapproval of disfavoured behaviours. Deregulation becomes a symbol of weakness that is often politically unpopular. Despite the political dimensions, public officials should give greater attention to the health effects of public policies.

The government, then, has many legal 'levers' designed to prevent injury and disease and promote the public's health. Legal interventions can be highly effective and need to be part of the public health officer's arsenal. However, legal interventions can be controversial, raising important ethical, social, constitutional, and political issues. These conflicts are complex, important, and fascinating for students of public health law.

4.5. Conclusion

> I desire, in closing this series of introductory papers, to leave one great fact clearly stated. There is no wealth but life. Life, including all its

powers of love, of joy, and of admiration. That country is richest which nourishes the greatest number of noble and happy human beings; that man is richest, who, having perfected the functions of his own life to the utmost, has also the widest helpful influence, both personal, and by possessions, over the lives of others.

(John Ruskin 1862)

Health is foundational to the functioning of societies as well as individuals. A broad understanding of 'the good' of population health and the role of government in its implementation is critical to the public health enterprise. In the late twentieth century scholars and politicians posed a key question: 'What desires and needs do you have as an autonomous, rights-bearing person to privacy, liberty, and free enterprise?' Now it is important to ask another kind of question, equally important to human well-being: 'In what kind of a community do you want and deserve to live, and what personal interests are you willing to forgo to achieve a good and healthful society?'

This chapter has proposed an action agenda to help attain healthier and safer populations:

- Create a new public health ethic in society that truly values the health and welfare of the people: advocate for a renewed commitment to the ideals of community and partnership, and stress citizens' duties to help and protect their fellow human beings.
- Help communities use law as a tool for health promotion and disease prevention: tax and spend to create incentives for healthy activities, alter the informational and built environments to reduce risk behaviours, lower economic disparities to improve morbidity and mortality, regulate for the public's welfare, pursue tort litigation to innovate for safety, and deregulate to reduce harm.

5

Population-Level Bioethics: Mapping a New Agenda

Daniel Wikler and Dan W. Brock

5.1. What is Distinctive in a Population Focus? A Bird's Eye Perspective in Bioethics

Bioethics was long focused on ethical issues arising in the relationships and interactions of individual patients and their physicians, as well as individual investigators and their research subjects. Ethical issues arising at the population level are no less acute, but are much less visible to lay people, to health professionals, and to many bioethicists. The issues come into focus only when one adopts a bird's eye view that looks at populations. From this perspective, new issues become visible, and their close kinship to long-debated ethical questions in other fields such as population policy, environmental health, and political philosophy becomes apparent. Even as investigation, debate, and education continue in the clinical settings in which bioethics has been most at home, an extensive, new, and largely unexplored region of bioethics is coming into view. The bird's eye perspective of this population level bioethics includes consideration not only of health care but also of other social determinants of health, including socio-economic standing, environmental and working conditions, and social exclusion. Its subject therefore is health rather than health care alone, insofar as health can be affected by conditions and interventions in any of these domains.

The focus of population-level bioethics is broader than bioethics at the clinical level not only for its concern with groups but also in that it is extended in both space and time. It extends naturally to a global focus, permitting population-level comparisons of the extent, direction, and distribution of health prospects. The least healthy populations, most of which are in developing countries, become especially prominent from this perspective; for them, the stakes are highest and the ethical dilemmas most severe. Population-level bioethics is also extended temporally, taking into account the consequences of present day events that affect the health of future generations, and their size and makeup. In so doing, it transcends disciplinary borders into demography, gerontology, genetics, and economic development.

Bioethics, as a normative discipline, draws on moral philosophy and other sources of reflection on values. But whereas clinical bioethics looks to the morality of individual conduct and character, population-level bioethics relies principally on theories of justice and other political philosophy. Where clinical bioethics speaks of the rights and responsibilities of patients and doctors, bioethics at the population level assesses the obligations of societies toward their members and each other and the norms governing complex relationships of individuals, groups, and the state.

All of these distinctive features of bioethics at the population level emerge from a brief survey of some of the outstanding issues. We will not explore here any of these issues in detail, but only suggest some of the key questions that need to be addressed within each issue. Our hope in surveying these issues is to supplement clinical bioethics by stimulating more work by bioethicists and others on these population level issues.

5.2. Society's Responsibility for Health

Most industrialized countries accept the World Health Organization's dictum that stewardship of health systems is a responsibility of national governments (WHO 2000b: 119f). For decades, the exception among developed countries was the United States. In the 1980s, the 'Washington Consensus' in developmental economics raised this perspective to the level of principle for developing countries (Williamson 1997), prompting states to privatize health care along with other basic services. Since then, seemingly inexorable increases in costs for health care have put pressure even on wealthy countries that have accepted health as a national responsibility, such as Canada, where the government's near-monopoly on health services has been a defining principle of national identity. At one time, social responsibility for health—either as a goal or as a reality—was a given among developed countries; the puzzle was American exceptionalism. Now, the debate is open throughout the world. What case can be made for the assumption of responsibility for health by the state (Szreter 1988)? What form should that responsibility take? To what extent can the extent of that responsibility be guided by moral argument and to what extent must it be determined by political consensus? What effects have recent privatization efforts had on the justice of health systems in which they have taken place?

5.3. Individual Responsibility for Health

Poor health and disability is not always a calamity that just happens to someone. We can increase our chances of staying healthy if we eat prudently, exercise, avoid tobacco and drugs, handle dangerous or toxic objects and substances with due caution, and comply with medical advice. Each of us takes chances sometimes, and some people become sick, disabled, or die as a result. What implications, if any, do these facts have for health policy and public health? Britain's National Health Service does not generally offer tattoo removal (Klein 1997; New 1997), but will remove birthmarks that disfigure to a similar degree. Yet the NHS, like public and private insurers everywhere, pay for treatment for smokers who contract lung cancer. But most are opposed. Should the health field find room for concepts of desert, fault, responsibility, and blame that are traditionally more at home in the courtroom? (Wikler 2004) What would be the distributive effects of doing so, and would the result be fairer, particularly in light of the fact that many unhealthy behaviors such as smoking and poor nutrition are disproportionately concentrated in lower socioeconomic classes (Roemer 1993, Lantz et al. 1998)? How would assignment of personal responsibility for health affect the moral norms underpinning the field of health promotion, and its inclusion on the agenda of public and international health agencies (Leichter 2003)? If assignment of personal responsibility should be relevant to various health policies, should it also be reflected in individual patient care decisions by physicians at the clinical level as well? Would it be consistent to give weight to personal responsibility at policy levels, but to ignore it in clinical contexts? What would be the ethical consequences of physicians assessing not just patients' needs for care, but also their responsibility for their health needs, in allocating their services? To the extent that health disparities can be traced to the imprudence of the poor, should this issue be regarded as a personal failing rather than as a social injustice (Barry 2005)?

5.4. Health and Human Rights: What Relation to Population-Level Bioethics?

The field of health and human rights is ubiquitous and official: it is recognized in international treaties,[1] and its practitioners are found in UN agencies and in much of the world. Some work in bioethics outside the United States also draws heavily on human rights, but in the United States bioethics remains an entirely separate academic specialization. The field of human rights is largely guided by lawyers, while bioethics looks to academic philosophy. The two fields overlap but little in personnel, journals,[2] or conferences. Yet at the population level they address many of the same issues, such as health care priority-setting, the ethics of research with human subjects, ethical limits on public health interventions that threaten civil liberties, and public participation in health policy. Is the de facto segregation of these fields an historical accident or is it based on a rational division of labor? Would it be useful to attempt to integrate these fields, or are they best left separate (Mann 1997, Mann et al. 1999)? How might they be effectively integrated? Is human rights theory potentially more useful for some areas of population-level bioethics than others, and if so which?

---

[1] See Office of High Commissioner for Human Rights (1976) International Covenant on Economic, Social and Cultural Rights, Article 12. Available at: http://193.194.138.190/html/menu3/b/a_cescr.htm (Accessed 5 May 2006).

[2] However, there are some exceptions, see, for example, *Health and Human Rights: An International Journal*. Boston: Harvard School of Public Health.

5.5. Priority Setting

Scarce resources require priority-setting: among treatments and interventions; among recipient populations; and in guiding research and training. These are often tragic choices. If treatment for AIDS is much less cost-effective than prevention (De Cock et al. 2002; Marseille et al. 2002), should funds be channeled to prevention even as needy patients suffer and die (Masaki et al. n.d.)? When treatment programs for AIDS lack enough money and doctors to treat everyone, should the sickest be first in priority, or should those who play essential social or medical roles such as teachers and health care workers receive priority (Macklin 2004)? And if so, should productive workers be favored over retirees? In the WHO's '3-by-5' program which aims to place 3 million patients with HIV/AIDS on anti-retroviral therapy by the end of 2005, how should those patients be selected from among the 6 million patients in need of therapy (Capron and Reis 2005)? If some patients are more expensive to reach and to treat, should they be abandoned in favor of patients cured more easily and cheaply? What do we need to know, or to develop, to address these moral questions? What role is there for moral reasoning, and what kind of contribution can ethics, and in particular theories of justice, make (Daniels 2005)? In general, should priorities in the health care system mirror choices individuals make or would make in buying insurance for themselves?

5.6. Cost-Effectiveness Analysis (CEA)

Cost-effective health interventions achieve the greatest health gains possible with the resources available. Cost-effectiveness analysis purports to offer evidence-based, objective guidance for priority-setting among health interventions, identifying those with the greatest potential health benefits given the resources available. But CEA is not value-free. On closer examinations, it is possible to identify moral assumptions that are embedded in CEA; and thereby to try to determine which of those assumptions are ethically defensible (Gold et al. 1996; Brock 2003a). For example, in a CEA one must decide whether to apply discount rates to future health benefits, as is routinely done to future costs and financial gains, and whether to give different value to health benefits for different age groups (Brock 2004a; Williams 1997).

The decision may have a strong effect on the relative priority given to acute versus preventive interventions and to interventions serving different age groups (Tsuchiya 2000). And what is the role of CEA in the moral and policy deliberation that results in prioritization for interventions (Murray et al. 2002)? A small but important literature, to which contributions have been made by philosophers, economists, and others, identifies a number of elements in CEA that represent substantive moral commitments. Influential guidance documents have urged CEA to be as value-free as possible, but some assumptions about values are probably ineliminable and should be made explicit (Menzel et al. 2002). CEA, moreover, does not offer a suitable guide for priority-setting unless it is joined by equity considerations. Those equity considerations need to be made explicit, together with the moral reasons for different positions on them, to help guide policy makers using CEAs. It is possible that equity considerations could be introduced as weights within the CEA, but it is not clear that this would be desirable, particularly in the face of widespread ethical disagreement about many of them.

5.7. Health Measurement

Individuals who submit to regularly-scheduled physical examinations can chart their health states over time. On the population level, data from many individuals is combined to yield a measure of population health (Murray et al. 2002). At the individual level, the data in the chart—blood pressure test scores, for example—may not in themselves represent any significant value judgments. 'Summary measures' of population health, however, cannot easily avoid them. An overall measure of population health incorporates data from many tests on many people and must assign weights to each in order to compute the whole. Our estimate of the health of a population, from this perspective, reflects our measurements of the prevalence of blindness and deafness; but it also reflects our judgments of the relative degree to which these two states detract from overall health. These judgments are typically derived from research on the preferences of the affected population, or of experts, and are therefore based on measurement as well. But these preferences may themselves involve value judgments. Moreover, the preferences of subgroups may vary considerably. A much-discussed example is the difference of views between disabled and non-disabled people regarding their disability (Brock 2000, 2003b). Blind people, for example, usually regard blindness to be less of a problem, relative to other health deficits, than sighted people do. The two groups would therefore differ in judging the contribution to population health of programs to prevent or cure blindness; and these differences would in turn affect the results of cost-effectiveness analyses of such interventions. In measuring population health, one must choose between relying on one or the other of these different sets of preferences, or else averaging or otherwise combining them, but each of these choices arguably embodies and reflects a particular set of values. A different alternative still is to abandon all preference-based measures in favor of an objective measure of health.

5.8. Health and Economic Development

One of Dr. Gro Harlem Brundtland's main objectives during her term of office as Director-General of the World Health Organization was to make health the concern not only of the health minister—often a lonely and embattled figure, perceived as a net absorber of funds—but also the ministers of finance and economic development. Her Commission on Macroeconomics and Health (2001), chaired by Jeffrey Sachs, coordinated the work of a small army of economists to make the case for health as an engine of economic development. But is there a less welcome suggestion implicit in this approach: that higher priority should be placed on health for the productive than for the elderly, the disabled, the uneducated, and others whose health care is unlikely to yield a positive return on social investment apart from the health benefit given to these individuals (Brock 2003b)? Likewise, this approach seems to imply a higher priority for health interventions that serve more productive individuals and groups (Donaldson 1999). This result is deeply in conflict with common norms of medicine that direct physicians to focus only on patients' needs and to ignore their social value or worth. These implications are not endorsed by WHO (nor by most others who make similar arguments for attaching high priority to health over other needs), but is this really consistent? And what follows if it is not?

5.9. Vulnerable Populations and Emergency Humanitarian Interventions

An encounter between doctor and patient in a pleasant suburban clinic may have little in common with the attempt by a volunteer physician to minister to the needs of refugees fleeing attempted genocide or desperate victims of a natural disaster. Resources in these emergency interventions are invariably stretched to the breaking point; both patients and health workers may be agitated and frightened; mutual distrust is commonplace, and there may be no source of legitimate authority (Lautze et al. 2004). Yet patients do not give up their rights in these emergency situations, nor physicians their professional obligations. For example, patients may be even more sensitive than usual about lapses of confidentiality about sensitive medical information. But it is not enough for health workers in emergency humanitarian interventions simply to reaffirm their commitment to conventional medical ethics. The unconventional context of care presents novel dilemmas that need to be thought out afresh. For example, physicians may feel strongly that those fleeing a genocide have a greater claim on their services than those perpetrating it (Tobin 2005). Such moral quandaries are exacerbated by the fragmentation of services as humanitarian agencies with diverse nationalities, goals, and modus operandi occupy the same physical space, with various levels of cooperation and competition. Should there be some common understandings of the moral rules? What should the rules be, and who should determine them?

5.10. Risks and the People Who Bear Them

In their recent broadside against cost-benefit analysis, Frank Ackerman and Lisa Heinzerling (2004) open with a telling anecdote. Two recent immigrants walking along the oceanfront in California died when struck by a car whose driver was chatting on a cell phone. The authors trace their demise to a decision by the California legislature not to ban the use of cell phones by drivers, which they say was influenced by studies that concluded that 'people who are talking while driving are willing to pay a lot to talk on the phone—more than many people who face deadly risks are willing to pay to avoid the risk of being killed.' The authors point out that no money, no compensation, actually changes hands. The rationale for the willingness-to-pay test is that it is welfare maximizing, but why should it matter that risk imposers are willing to pay more than risk avoiders if no compensation is ever made to those who suffer the risk? The pedestrians end up in the morgue; was this result fair to them? Moreover, willingness to pay to avoid risks is strongly influenced by ability to pay, and so by inequalities in wealth, which are often unjust inequalities. Clearly, there is a moral calculus at work in these analyses, one that influences the health of populations. Is the authors' example telling, or is it a distortion of the way that these analyses are applied to health-related policy decisions? And whatever the moral calculations actually amount to, are they justified? If the 'willingness to pay test' is not an ethically acceptable standard for risk imposition, what would be (Wolff forthcoming)?

5.11. Environmental Equity

Some people will pay a lot to avoid living near toxic waste dumps, or in housing with high levels of lead paint, or in a flood plain. Many more would like to, but do not have the money; as a result, they are more likely to become sick. Moreover, wealthier people have a double advantage, since they are more likely to be well-educated and to know what and where the hazards are, and how to avoid them. Consequently, exposure to environmental health hazards is by no means uniform across the population. The inequity is greater still when the toxins that put some at risk result from decisions by firms to benefit their investors by skimping on pollution controls. Should these disparities be understood merely as yet another reason it is bad to be poor, or is there a special, distinctive, and urgent reason for attempting to achieve a more equitable pattern of immunity from environmental threats to health, even as economic and other disparities persist? Do the health effects of economic disparities have any special moral importance, and if so why and what are its implications for public policy (O'Neill et al. 2003; Levy et al. 2006)?

5.12. Populations and Genes

A century ago, the prospect of 'improving' human heredity animated scientists, officials, and lay enthusiasts who flocked to the eugenics movement (Paul 1995). In the wake of Nazi barbarities associated with eugenics, it has become impolitic to speak openly about improving population health and well-being by trying to influence the kinds of people who will be born. But is this goal in fact ethically unacceptable if dissociated with other immoral features of many historical eugenics programs (Buchanan et al. 2000)? New reproductive methods present some choice among potential offspring, and more choices lie just over the horizon. No one favors a return of the coercive and punitive aspects of the old eugenics, but what of the movement's positive goals? Are they implicit in some health programs, such as genetic screening and testing or preimplantation genetic diagnosis that wear other labels (Wikler 1999)? If so, should they be reined in? Or can we learn from the history of the eugenics movement what safeguards must be in place to protect individual rights if we are to pursue goals of population-level genetic health (Wasserman et al. 2005)? What goals, values and standards would we be discussing seriously at this point in this era of rapid development of genetics and associated sciences if we did not have this bogey to contend with?

5.13. Protecting Health, Endangering Civil Liberties

Conventional wisdom had only recently assured us infectious disease was a threat only to people in the poorest countries, or those who traveled there. But then came AIDS; and after that SARS; and we are now bracing ourselves for a pandemic of avian flu. AIDS and SARS tested public health protections and, in many countries, found them wanting. We now know better than to let our guard down. But is it possible to be *too* prepared (Sunstein 2005)? What are the costs—monetary, social, legal, ethical, and psychological—of giving priority to containing outbreaks of infectious disease? Hong Kong health authorities complain today of 'collateral damage' from the SARS outbreak, as resources are rechanneled from other needed services to guard against any threat of a new outbreak. The prospect of bioterrorism sets nations further on edge. The first price to be paid in the event of an outbreak of an uncontrollable infectious disease, however, may be our civil liberties. In the face of potential panic, how secure are these freedoms, and how secure should they be (Gostin 2002a)? What sacrifices might be justified to guard health? And what sacrifices might be justified not to guard health, but to reassure the public? What lesson should other countries learn from Cuba's success in limiting the spread of HIV by interning HIV-positive citizens (Bayer and Healton 1989; Scheper-Hughes 1993)? Does the threat of epidemic trump all other considerations? And what if we have entered an era in which we are never entirely free of such a threat? Threats from a time-limited epidemic may at least be seen as only requiring temporary suspensions of civil liberties. But if fears of bioterrorism become permanent features of the landscape, will steps to combat bioterrorism result in permanent erosion of important civil liberties (Kellman 2001; Annas 2002)?

5.14. Global Aging

In both developed and developing countries the most profound demographic change in this century will be the aging of the population. Since older people tend to need more health services, this trend will put new stresses on health systems (WHO 2002a). The inversion of the population pyramid, with elderly dependents looking for support from a narrowing base of productive younger people, will have ripple effects throughout society. As the number of old people rises sharply, will the cost of their care deprive younger people of their rightful standard of living (WHO 2002b)? Does equity require that countries facing the greatest age imbalance begin to limit the expectations of their older citizens? Should there be standards of equitable sharing of health resources between age cohorts, and if so how can these be established (Daniels 1998; WHO 2003)? When do limits on those resources constitute unjust age discrimination (Brock 1989)? A fundamental question of justice in the health sector in this century will be how resources should be distributed to different age groups.

5.15. Global Health Equity

The biggest difference between growing up in a developing country and being a child in a rich country, it has been observed, is the experience of frequent serious illness and the ever present specter of death. The burden of disease falls disproportionately on the billions of human beings, of all ages, who make up the poor majority of the poorest countries. Which of these inequalities are inequitable (Temkin 1993, Lynch et al. 1998)? Why? Are global health disparities unjust only if they can be traced to unjust causes—to colonialism and imperialism, to unequal leverage over tariffs, quotas, and other terms of trade, to monopoly powers enjoyed by first-world based food and drug companies, and to the long-term effects of proxy wars instigated by the Great Powers (Pogge 2002)? How much of the disparities in health and longevity among nations can be traced to one of these injustices? Can we distinguish health disparities that result from such injustices from other 'natural' disparities? Are there other moral grounds for condemning these disparities even when they appear not to result from injustices (Risse 2005)? And is there any reason for singling out disparities in health among the myriad effects of greater poverty? Whatever our answer to these questions, what would constitute redress?

5.16. Inequalities in Health Within Countries

Inequalities in health within national boundaries are much greater than most people realize, and they are strongly linked to socioeconomic status. For example, the difference in life expectancies between counties in the United States with the worst poverty and the highest inequality compared with counties with the highest incomes and least inequality is greater than the mortality effects of lung cancer, diabetes, motor vehicle crashes, HIV/AIDS, suicide, and homicide (Pappas et al. 1993; Murray et al. 1998). For many of us, these inequalities seem to be prima facie evidence of injustice; indeed to constitute an injustice in themselves. But on what ethical basis does this intuition rest? As with health disparities between countries, we must ask whether all health inequalities within a country are unjust, as much of the health policy literature seems to assume (Marchand et al. 1998; Daniels et al. 2000b)? Is it unjust, for example, that women outlive men in most countries (Kekes 1997)? When are health inequalities inequities, and why? What patterns of inequality in health are the most objectionable from a moral point of view, and what kinds of changes in the distribution of health states and prospects best resolves them? Should concern for equity in health focus on inequalities between individuals or between groups, and if the latter which groups (Murray et al. 1999; Braveman et al. 2001; Asada and Hedemann 2002; Gakidou and King 2002)? Should economists' measures of income inequality, such as the Gini coefficient or the Atkinson/Kolm measure (Atkinson 1970) be taken over to the field of health without revision, and if so which is the most germane to ethical concerns (Lecluyese and Cleemput 2005; Low and Low 2006)? And what, precisely, is the objectionable feature of health disparities—the gap itself, or the poor health of the worst-off (Marchand and Wikler 2002)? Should we give lower priority to health interventions that tend to benefit healthier people, even if they are more cost-effective? How should we try to balance the goals of maximizing and equalizing population health?

5.17. Social Determinants of Population Health

A burgeoning body of research in recent decades has demonstrated the profound impact on population health and health inequalities of social conditions such as education and literacy, socio-economic inequality, social control and supports, and a wide array of social policies concerning transportation, housing, unemployment, and so forth (Marmot 2004). Indeed, together with the effects of traditional public health measures such as clean water supplies and immunization programs, these have greater impacts on health and health inequalities than do health care and inequalities in access to health care. Traditional philosophical work in theories of justice has addressed these social determinants without adequate recognition of their impact on health. To what extent—if at all—must theories of justice that address non-health domains be revised in light of our new understanding of how these domains affect health? And if they should be revised, how should they be revised? What weight should be given to the differential health impacts of social policy in such fields as education, transportation and housing? Should we seek to require health impact assessments of policies in these domains, similar to the environmental impact assessments now often required (Levy et al. 2006)?

5.18. Practice Implications of a Population Perspective

Geoffrey Rose, the British epidemiologist, contrasted the 'medical' and 'population' approaches to hypertension and other risk factors that are major determinants of population health (Rose 1985). The medical strategy is to identify the high-risk individuals and treat them so as to head off their impending health problems. The population approach instead seeks to reduce the risks of the population as a whole, usually by non-individual and non-medical interventions. For example, while the medical approach would provide drugs for hypertension to the worst cases, the population approach would work toward a reduction in the salt content of processed foods, lowering everyone's risk and thereby the number of deaths attributable to hypertension. While these approaches might be complementary, they have not received equal emphasis or funding. Should the choice between them be based on cost-effectiveness grounds, or are there other moral issues at stake? Is the medical approach more respectful of individual choice by leaving individuals free to determine what responses to risk factors for disease are appropriate for them? Or is the population approach more equitable in that it benefits even those who are not aware of their health needs or who are unable to seek care? Does the population approach impose an intervention on some members of the population who may not be significantly at risk, and if so is this an important objection to them? Does the population approach distribute its benefits more equitably by seeking to reduce the risk factor equally for all? Which is more likely to contribute to the 'medicalization' of everyday life; and why should we be concerned if it does? What considerations should determine the relative emphasis given to the medical and population approaches for specific health risks?

5.19. Research Ethics and Social Justice

Developing countries offer advantages to scientists and pharmaceutical firms seeking test sites for new drugs and therapies. Participants' bodies in these countries are less likely to be carrying other drugs that could confuse outcomes of trials. Higher incidence of many diseases places an adequate supply of potential participants at the hospital door so that trials can get underway quickly. Costs are often lower and regulation less strict. These advantages for sponsors and scientists, however, reflect vulnerabilities in the host population. What moral rules should govern the contract between scientists (and their sponsors) and participants in these developing-country experiments (Brock and Wikler 2006)? Is it permissible to test products that offer little or no medical benefit to the local population, such as a malaria vaccination offering tourists a few days' immunity? Can other benefits such as strengthening the health care infrastructure compensate for a lack of medical benefit? What should be the standard of care offered to participants, including those serving as controls? In particular, when other treatments have been proven effective should controls be given those treatments even when they are not available or affordable in the local setting, or may placebo controls or less than the best treatments be used? How should participants in trials in developing countries be fairly selected? Does the sponsor owe the participants or the broader community in which the trial takes place access to treatments proven effective in these trials, and if so for how long? Do they owe anything further to the community? Who would be the loser if stringent requirements along these lines were imposed and the developing-country sites became less attractive to sponsors as a result? And is this likely to happen?

5.20. Health System Reform

While health systems have contributed to the remarkable rise in longevity enjoyed throughout the world until the AIDS pandemic, they remain inadequate to the demands placed on them. Lack of money, trained health workers, and management expertise hobble health systems in much of the developing world, even as AIDS and other emerging diseases increase the need for effective treatment. Changes in the structure, financing, and management of health systems might permit these health systems to deliver more, or deliver it more equitably, without increases in state funding, and we live in an era of unprecedented experimentation. But not all changes are improvements, even if they are labeled 'reforms.' Are there norms that might guide health system reform so that it becomes (or remains) just? Can we specify procedural requirements on health system reform, such as public participation, transparency, and the availability of grievance procedures (Daniels et al. 1996)? And should substantive rules be specified as well, such as reducing gender, racial or ethnic discrimination, or giving special concern for the poor and other vulnerable individuals or groups (Mackenbach 2004)? Which health system reform efforts should be regarded as positive and negative models, respectively? What are the positive and negative effects of various forms of privatization within health care systems taking place around the world today?

5.21. Conclusion

The population-level ethical issues surveyed in this brief account could hardly have greater importance for us as individuals, as citizens of our countries, and as a species. Even after several decades of debate over bioethics, however, debate has only barely begun on most of these questions. Why have the ethical questions with the greatest scope and impact been investigated the least? The answer is largely historical. One source for bioethics is the code of conduct of medical professionals; another is the patients' rights movement of the 1960s and later. Both of these spoke to the experience of individual doctors and patients. Population-level ethical issues in bioethics are usually invisible at this level. There has been a corresponding difference in the receptivity of the professional groups involved. While medical professionals may have opened ethical debates to patients and their advocates only grudgingly at first, these discussions have now transcended professional boundaries and are understood as issues that are of interest to everyone. Economists, demographers, and epidemiologists who work on population health focused on the scientific issues in their work; indeed, as we have pointed out, the pressing ethical questions were often not identified as such. In any case, they were unaccustomed to seeking to engage bioethicists in discussions of the ethical dilemmas they encountered; for one thing, there were very few bioethicists prepared to be engaged.

But all this is, or should be, history. The issues are in view. Though still small, a promising literature has been created. Bioethics training programs have, in a few places, begun to incorporate or even emphasize population-level issues. And a growing number of scientists, managers, officials, and others concerned with population health have had useful encounters with these discussions. Some of them may become motivated to becoming ethicists themselves.

We reiterate that our aim in this chapter has been to sketch out a research agenda for a population level bioethics to supplement the traditional focus of clinical bioethics. The latter remains important to each of us in our roles as health professionals, patients, and citizens. But the issues arising at the population level are no less grave, and though their impact on our lives as individuals is often invisible to us, it is often profound. They also help to determine which choices are available to doctors and patients in the clinic. An expansion of the field of bioethics to the population level will illuminate the traditional arena of the field while engaging, after a period of relative neglect, a host of issues of front-rank human importance.

6

Parental Choice and Expert Knowledge in the Debate about MMR and Autism

Tom Sorell

In democracies, conflicts between public opinion and expert opinion can be morally and politically charged. It is one thing for the public to be alienated from expert aesthetic opinion, as when millions in public funds are spent on an 'artwork' that ordinary observers dislike; in that sort of case, although the 'artwork' can appear to be to a waste of money, it is widely accepted, even by the general public, that aesthetic taste varies, and that different works of art should get exposure, even if they are unpopular. It is widely accepted, too, that exposure to new works widens aesthetic taste, rather than contributing to its deterioration. It is quite another matter where expert opinion supports a coercive policy that the public, or sections of the public, resist. Especially where the policy is introduced for the good of the public, the resistance quickly invites the question of who is a better judge of the public good than the public itself. It is hard to confront this question without appearing either paternalistic or relativistic. I shall argue that where the coercive policy is backed by a clear medical consensus, appropriately reconsidered in the light of claims of doubters, there is sometimes a moral obligation on the part of the public to defer to the experts. The argument will be geared to the continuing controversy in the UK over the safety of the measles/mumps/rubella (MMR) vaccine. The vaccine is administered to children twice, at the ages of one and four. It was introduced into the UK in 1988, before which there was a separate vaccination for each of the three diseases.

6.1. MMR Vaccination after the Wakefield Paper

In 1998, Andrew Wakefield, a consultant gastroenterologist at the Royal Free Hospital in London, published with colleagues a paper in the *Lancet* suggesting that there was a link between the MMR vaccine and both bowel disease and autism in young children (Wakefield et al. 1998). Widespread publicity for this suggestion had the effect of reducing uptake of the MMR vaccine in Britain, and of increasing demand on the part of parents for separate vaccinations for measles, mumps and rubella. A pressure group of parents of children who are believed to have been harmed by vaccinations in the UK—JABS—has also been active in making representations against the triple vaccine.[1] The NHS has resisted a change of vaccination policy, and the reduced uptake for the combined MMR vaccine has led to an increase in the incidence of measles. In Scotland, for example, cases of measles and mumps have risen markedly up to and including 2006.[2]

Recently, some of the co-authors with Wakefield of the 1998 paper have repudiated its results. So has the *Lancet*. Many scientific re-examinations of the evidence have taken place since 1998, and they, too have largely disagreed with Wakefield (Institute of Medicine 2004). Wakefield himself has stuck by his findings.[3]

The most obvious question that arises from the MMR controversy is, 'Who is right?' *Does* the vaccine increase the risk of bowel disease or autism, or doesn't it? Only those with relevant medical expertise are in a position to answer, and they do not all agree. Still, there is a clear consensus among them to the effect that Wakefield's claims are doubtful, and that the MMR vaccine should go on being administered. However, given that the UK government cannot *prove* that the MMR vaccine is safe, shouldn't the triple vaccine be withdrawn

---

[1] JABS: Justice Awareness and Basic Support. Available at: http://www.jabs.org.uk

[2] See http://news.scotsman.com/scotland.cfm?id=2305852005 (accessed 28 March 2006).

[3] For the various statements of editors, Wakefield and co-authors see *Lancet* (2004) 363: 820–4.

for the time being, or replaced for the time being with single vaccinations, as Wakefield and the JABS pressure group urge? This issue is one of a range that arise when there is a conflict between popular opinion and expert opinion in a democracy. I shall argue that the burden of proof is on Wakefield and his supporters to show that there should be a departure from the established policy. Peer review of Wakefield's study has not produced general agreement to his findings on the part of those scientists who have tested them. On the contrary, scepticism has been the much more usual reaction. UK public health bodies have therefore been reasonable to resist a change of vaccination policy on the balance of the available evidence. Indeed, they have been more than reasonable, having gone to considerable trouble to follow up any UK cases which *prima facie* favour the Wakefield hypothesis. Many of these cases turn out to be explicable in ways that do not call in question the MMR vaccine.

Although Wakefield and his supporters have turned up evidence that requires explanation, this evidence does not begin to indicate that the danger of MMR outweighs its benefits. Nor does it seem to be true that a reversion to separate vaccines would be more beneficial, all things considered, than continuing to offer the triple vaccine. The fact that many *parents* prefer the single vaccine has no particular weight unless the MMR vaccine just is, for independent medical reasons, inferior to the single vaccines. In the MMR case, I want to argue, parental opinion is no more relevant than public opinion in general, since what matters is the actual effects of the MMR vaccine, which is not a matter settled by public opinion or common sense, and that is all that most parents or most of the public can bring to bear. It is true that parents have a responsibility, both legal and moral, for their children's health, but that does not mean that they can always discharge the responsibility without deferring to expert opinion. In the MMR case, this deference is in order, especially when the experts have gone to so much trouble to investigate lay suspicions of a link between MMR and childhood disorders.

6.2. Respect for Parents and Patients

A good way of broaching the issues raised by MMR is against the background of a debate held at the annual conference of the British Medical Association in Bournemouth, in July 2001. There a motion proposing that single vaccines be made available by the NHS was put to the vote. Opponents of the motion said that single vaccines were not as effective as the triple vaccine, and that allowing people to have their children separately vaccinated would reduce the rate of immunization even further, at a time when levels of immunization in the UK were below those recommended by the World Health Organization.[4]

The motion was overwhelmingly defeated. One of its supporters, Dr Ian Robbe, senior lecturer in public health at the University of Wales, Cardiff, was quoted as saying, 'This is about the issue of respect that I offer as a doctor to a parent or patient. The evidence on MMR is very mixed. I think not to respect the parents' position is not to give people the right to make a choice—it is taking choice away from them.'[5] Robbe's position combines a number of views that are tempting to adopt, but I think wrong to adopt, in relation to MMR. The issue is precisely *not* one of respect. It is to do with the state of the evidence about the effects of MMR and the risks of having a different scheme of vaccination. Those who are able to, can speak to the relevant effects and risks. Presumably Robbe can. Presumably he is an expert who agrees that single vaccinations ought to be made available. But those who disagree with that policy on scientific grounds do not show disrespect for Robbe, and those who disagree on the same grounds with parents do not show them disrespect either. The experts *would* be showing disrespect if they disagreed with parents on non-scientific grounds—say on the basis that they detest the behaviour of the children brought up by these parents and have contempt for the parents. But they do not show disrespect simply by disagreeing. Nor is disrespect shown by distinguishing between lay opinion and expert opinion in the MMR debate. Nor, finally, is any disrespect shown by supposing that expert opinion carries more weight in this case than lay opinion. I enlarge on this point later.

Robbe seems to me wrongly to transfer to the MMR case a way of thinking about the doctor–patient relationship that leaves out the public health aspects of MMR and leaves out the fact that it affects people—children—other than those making decisions about vaccination. Let us begin with the standard doctor–patient relationship. If there is a disagreement between an adult patient and a doctor over the patient's

[4] http://news.bbc.co.uk/1/hi/in_depth/health/2001/bma_conference/1424527.stm (accessed 28 March 2006).

[5] Ibidem.

health, it is plausible to many people to say that it is for the patient to choose even if one of the patient's options is to ignore advice that objectively would benefit him. Not to leave the choice to the patient would be a way of denying his autonomy. And as soon as weight is given to autonomy, then so must weight be given to choices that treat health improvement as only one desirable thing among others, and one that can be outweighed by others in a patient's scheme of values. Again, if the patient autonomously makes a medically inadvisable decision, he takes the consequences. It's his health, his life and making a decision that is medically disadvantageous for him will not harm anyone else, at least on many occasions. Of course, in some cases involving adults who decide to ignore good medical advice, public health can also be affected. But Robbe is evidently not thinking of these cases when he says that refusing choice is a form of disrespect. If an autonomous adult is discovered to have a contagious disease and refuses treatment, or refuses to take steps to limit his contacts with others, it is not disrespecting the patient to argue with him on public health grounds, or to refuse him the choice of infecting others.[6] Choosing to infect others is not one of the choices protected by a duty of respect for patients. Nor is it a choice protected by a duty of respect for parents when parents are deciding on medical treatment for their children. In the MMR case, parents' decisions to forgo vaccination or to take single vaccinations can affect the level of immunization of everyone else. So it is never the parents alone who take the consequences of a bad decision.[7] Parents have a responsibility to have their children vaccinated against measles, mumps and rubella,[8] and they are understandably reluctant to do so in an atmosphere where the safety of vaccinations seems to be in doubt. One reason why parental reluctance might be weighty in cases other than MMR is that parents typically love

---

[6] Even in cases where the medical effects of ignoring undisputed medical advice fall mainly on the patient, there can be other bad effects on the doctor or the health service. It is not disrespecting a patient to ask him to take responsibility for some of these effects. On the contrary, it is paternalistic not to. For more in this vein, see Draper and Sorell (2002).

[7] Just how much is being risked depends on how many defect from the vaccination scheme. In a population where there were few defectors, the consequences of withdrawing one's children from the vaccination might be negligible, but this method of avoiding risk depends on free-riding on the decisions of other parents.

[8] The ground for this duty is complex. It derives from the duty to protect their children from the measles, mumps and rubella of others, *and* to limit the sources of infection of other people. Getting a vaccine in the context of an immunization programme satisfies both duties.

their children and can be assumed to give more weight to their children's interests than anyone else does, including the medical authorities. This is why their opinion about treatment is so important, and why getting it can be tantamount to giving the child's point of view the maximum influence in decisions where they cannot participate themselves. But the fact that parents are natural spokesmen for their children because they love their children is easily misinterpreted in the MMR case.

The fact that parents love their children makes it highly probable that they will not knowingly harm their children, and that they will actively help their children. But not knowingly harming one's children is compatible with harming them unwittingly, through lack of relevant knowledge. Similarly, actively helping one's children is only going to be successful within the limits of one's competence. If you are lousy at maths, then no matter how conscientiously you try to help your children with their maths homework, it is not going to do them any mathematical good. In short, it is not true that everything that their children need is, or can be, provided by parents, even if the parents put their children's interests first. There is a division of labour, geared in part to expert knowledge. Parents entrust the health of their children to doctors, and usually do not educate their children themselves. If their children travel, parents often put their children's lives in the hands of car drivers or bus drivers and airline pilots. Independent authorities certify these people as competent, and it would be jeopardising the welfare of children if everyone regularly decided to take over piloting, doctoring, or education of their offspring themselves. When a pressure group or individual parents decide that single vaccinations would do just as well as the triple vaccine, however, they are precisely taking over the doctoring role from the doctors. And they should no more take over the role of doctor when they are not medically trained than they should entrust their house to questionable DIY skills when they can call on the services of a good builder. The fact that they love their house more than anyone else does not mean that they are competent to maintain it, and the fact that they love their child more than anyone else does not mean that they are always the best judge of medical treatment either.

Admittedly, there is a difference between the case where there is no medical consensus about a particular treatment and the MMR case. A parent discharges his responsibility for the health of his child by making himself or herself as well informed as possible and acting on the information, but sometimes the best information will not be good enough for a clear choice, because medical opinion itself is divided. In the MMR case, however, this does not appear to be so. The MMR vaccine is used worldwide, including in countries where the costs of medical negligence are very high and risks are not taken in the least casually; and there is wide agreement, even among the critics, that most people feel no ill effects from vaccinations, including MMR vaccinations. So we do not have an evenly balanced controversy tipping gradually in the direction of the conclusion that MMR is safe. Rather, it has always been the case that the evidence *against* the safety of MMR has been slight. Indeed, Wakefield's 1998 article turns out to have been much more tentative in its criticism of MMR than the tabloid newspapers that purported to report its conclusions.[9]

Parents can be forgiven for succumbing to the scare created by the tabloids, but because the issue is not *only* one of their child's health, and because the effectiveness of vaccinations in particular do depend on a very large take-up of injections, the consideration that not getting their children injected with the MMR vaccine was playing it safe for their children was not the only morally relevant consideration. Combined with the fact that the government went to some trouble to come out unequivocally in favour of MMR, that this message was overwhelmingly endorsed by GPs, and that actual doubts about MMR were raised fairly cautiously, it was probably not discharging one's responsibility to give more credence to JABS, Wakefield, or the newspapers.

6.3. Parental Choice, Realism and Deference to Experts

Even if there is a medical consensus about the safety of MMR and other vaccines, there are some who will say that it is only a consensus among practitioners of establishment medicine. It is possible to have unorthodox

---

[9] The Science Museum in London has put together for public consumption a very good and accessible summary of the scientific disagreements over MMR and the course of the controversy. See: http://www.sciencemuseum.org.uk/antenna/mmr/cip2/index.asp (accessed 28 March 2006). One important aspect of the controversy left out by both the Science Museum and by the present article is the role of the popular press in stirring up the MMR scare.

views about wellness as a patient; perhaps these deserve to be given weight in decisions about vaccination for one's children. This is the line of thought developed by Healthy Child Online, an American internet site promoting holistic medicine. On a web page devoted to vaccines, Healthy Child Online says the following:

Universal Vaccines for Everyone?

Does it make sense to mandate vaccines for every child given the risks involved? The public health strategy for eliminating diseases includes universal vaccines for everyone, regardless of risks to the individual. Some children must be sacrificed in order to achieve the goal of eradicating disease in a population. They tell us that more lives will be lost to the disease if we don't vaccinate against it. But is this statement really true in the current reality of high-tech medicine in a population with effective sanitation and knowledge about the immunology of breastfeeding?

We cannot wipe out every disease on the planet. It may be more sensible to focus on *strengthening* our children's immune systems to deal with the increasing number of different 'superbugs' created by the inappropriate and massive use of antibiotics than to inject numerous toxins into their delicate, developing bodies. If we use breastmilk, good nutrition, herbs, naturopathy, homoeopathy, or other immune-enhancing methods to keep our children's immune systems strong, then why would we want to inject foreign material and toxins into their bodies, especially since there have been no long term studies done to prove their safety? An increasing number of parents are not willing to take the risk of sacrificing their child to a point of view that goes against their core beliefs about health and wellness.

Parents Do Have A Choice

At the doctor's office, parents are given a two-page 'Vaccine Information Statement' which highlights the importance of vaccines and downplays the harmful effects. Many parents are coerced into vaccinating their children with the threat of losing their doctor, having their children denied school attendance, and charges of medical neglect. Children have actually been taken away from their parents, forcibly vaccinated, and placed in the care of the 'state' when their parents chose to protect them from vaccines. Informed consent means that an informed patient (or parent) should always have absolute freedom to accept or reject any specific medical treatment or procedure. The patient (or parent) has the right to be treated sensitively and compassionately while learning about his or her options. The doctor is both ethically obligated and legally required to participate in a communication process that helps the patient to understand risks and benefits as well as alternatives. There are informed consent statutes and case laws in all 50 states in the U.S. Why don't these revered informed consent laws apply when it comes to vaccines? Parents are almost never told about exemptions to state vaccine laws. They are usually told they do not have a choice.[10]

This statement puts forward its own (as far as I can tell) unsupported theory about how to strengthen the immune systems of children, and claims that its methods are superior to conventional ones in that they do not aim at universality and do not put foreign materials and toxins into children's bodies. The fact that what are normally toxins can sometimes help patients, and the fact that naturopathy and homeopathy are badly understood, are not acknowledged. Again, the fact that conventional medicine challenges some parents' core beliefs is taken to count against conventional medicine when what is ostensibly under discussion is what methods of immunization are safest and most effective—*whatever* parents' core beliefs are.

Healthy Child Online begs the question of whether vaccines are in fact safe when they assert that some parents choose to 'protect' their children from vaccines. Talk of protection implies, without establishing, that vaccines are harmful. Like Robbe, Healthy Child Online treats as interchangeable the question of a patient's right to choose for himself—disputable in any case where a patient's choice poses a public health risk—and a parent's right to choose for a child. And Healthy Child Online confuses the issue of what harms or benefits children by talking about the coercion of parents. Coercion is of course best avoided; but sometimes it is moral obligatory. It is not always against the medical and other interests of the child, as when parents addicted to drugs are forced to go onto a rehabilitation programme or else lose the children they are neglecting.

Let us leave aside cases in which there is significant disagreement among the experts over the correct medical treatment of a child. Let us concentrate on cases in which the experts agree amongst themselves, but the parents don't agree with the experts. Why, in that sort of case, is there *any* room morally for parents to choose or to affect the decision about treatment? One general reason for parents always having a say, even if it is not a decisive say, is that it is they who have the responsibility, outside episodes of medical treatment, for the care of the child. Parents are obliged to see to all of the needs of the child that they are aware of, including minor illnesses. They also have a role when doctors are involved, being expected to see that medication is administered,

[10] See: http://www.healthychild.com/database/vaccinations_a_parent_s_right_to_choose.htm (accessed 28 March 2006).

and they are relied upon to supply early warning of the need for medical interventions, including pubic health interventions. The control of head-lice is routinely privatized in this way, albeit with mixed results. Again, parents have responsibilities for, as it were, the whole child. The child's needs for food, water, shelter, education, protection from assault, transportation, entertainment, affection—all of these fall on parents, who are assumed, usually correctly, to be willing and able to meet those needs or to be able to identify others who can. Differently, parents are relied upon by the state to be local forces against offending behaviour. In relation to many of these duties, parents are in a sort of tacit partnership with professionals and officials: teachers, doctors, the police and so on. The presumption that the efforts of parents and public officials are directed to the same goals over a wide range of the needs of the very young justifies co-operation, and also consultation with parents when public officials and professionals see a need of the child that the parents do not.

The presumption that professionals, officials and parents are all on the same side in seeing to the needs of children does not mean that there can never be disagreements. After all, parents disagree amongst themselves, not only across families, but within families, about how the needs of the children should be met. In many cases these disagreements about needs stand alongside disagreements about the fine detail of upbringing and behaviour. And in many of these disagreements there may be no telling who is right, and no need to decide who is right in any case. There are many different variations on family life, and many of them are harmless and able to co-exist.

Some styles of family life can rub off on other families. Reflective parents observe how others raise children and sometimes wonder whether they do it well themselves. People from different generations in an extended family volunteer their opinions as well, often with a sense of its being important to do things one way rather than another. But it is mostly left to families themselves to develop their preferred practices for seeing to the needs of children. If they copy the practices of other families or listen to advice from relations, that is their choice. If they read parenting magazines and books and follow the advice they give, that is their decision, too. This is the large background against which it can seem presumptuous for people outside a family, or people other than parents, even to *comment* on how parents organize their children, unless that comment is asked for. It is against the same background that it can seem outrageous for an outsider to *insist* that parents do something for or to their children that those parents disagree with.

It takes something like the philosophical position called Realism to make sense of the possible appropriateness of outside interventions, especially those verging on or amounting to coercion. The key to Realism can be found in the common saying that believing doesn't make it so. We can believe things very firmly and sincerely—about many different topics—and be wrong despite the fact that we firmly and sincerely believe them. In particular, we are fallible—able to be wrong—about our states of health. It is possible to think that one has a disease and not have it, and possible to have a disease while believing one doesn't. It is also possible to be wrong about the effects on us of food we ingest, of things in the atmosphere, of failing to take exercise, and so on. These facts about our fallibility are not in the least affected by how *many* people believe a thing firmly or sincerely. Believing doesn't make it so, whether it's one person believing or millions. Instead there has to be something that makes a thing true, *independently* of its being believed—at least for many things we hold beliefs about.

It is not only possible but *easy* to be wrong about medical matters, just as it is not only possible but easy to be wrong about any subject matter in which understanding depends on principles about microstructures in organic or inorganic bodies. These are the principles taught in a medical education but not in what is called the university of life. And it is the existence of such principles that creates a big gap between expert knowledge in medicine or physics, say, and common sense or common opinion. There are other kinds of supposed expert knowledge—the knowledge of management consultants, say, or of lawyers—that does not depend on anything like these principles, and though people are able to make mistakes in law or in management, it is not because they are ignorant of the behaviour of organic or inorganic microstructures. In other words, there a kinds of expert knowledge that do not amount to *science*, where what counts as science is determined in part by comparability with physics or molecular biology.

One reason that medical expertise trumps other kinds of expertise, including homeopathic expertise—is that medicine *is* a science, or, probably better, a set of sciences. It explains and predicts a lot of effects with a reasonable small set of conceptually uniform principles supported by exact measurements. It is again on account of this scientific status that medicine trumps ordinary public or parental opinion, even where there exists a convention that parents are responsible for giving some of the medical care their children receive. It takes a very sophisticated (and in my view quite unfounded) philosophy of science to argue that medicine is no more authoritative than homoeopathy. And it takes a false philosophy of science again to show that medicine is not a science in any sense of 'science' that deserves to have authority, so that homeopathy is just as authoritative or common sense is just as authoritative.

Though the philosophy of science I favour supports deference to 'science' where it deserves the name, and where it is reflected in public policy, it does not support deference to every kind of professional regarded as an expert. It supports deference to public health officials who say that the MMR vaccine is safe; but it does not support deference to those who say that e.g. there should be an internal market in public medical provision, supply-side economics not being on a par as a science with molecular biology.

Are the grounds for deference in the MMR case also grounds for compelling parents who, on account of false or ill-founded 'core-beliefs', refuse to vaccinate their children? I think the answer is 'Yes', so long as every effort has been made first to explain the scientific basis for the need to vaccinate, this effort being directed at obtaining consent from the parents. But the policy described by Healthy Child Online of prohibiting school attendance and even of withdrawing the medical advice that the parents are ignoring at a risk to the public seem defensible if all else fails. On the other hand, removing the children altogether from the care of the parents, other things being equal, seems wildly disproportionate.

6.4. Expert Knowledge and Democracy

In the UK, the MMR scare inevitably has a political dimension. The Health Service is government-run and funded, and its policy is to administer the triple vaccine. Were there to be a scare over vaccines in general on the part of a large number of voters, vaccination policy would start to enter general political debate and party political campaigning. Suppose that there were a majority for withdrawing the MMR vaccine or some other vaccine or vaccinations in general. Would *that* be an argument for withdrawing the MMR vaccine or altering vaccination policy in some other way? Although it may sound anti-democratic to say so, my answer is that that would *not* by itself be an argument. The fact that a lot of medically inexpert people want a medical policy changed is only a reason for changing the medical policy if there are good reasons for changing the policy independently of how many people want it changed.

Once again what is at issue is the authority of expert knowledge where expert knowledge is relevant to a matter of public policy. The problem would not arise if expert medical knowledge in general, or knowledge or vaccines in particular, were widely distributed among the public. But public understanding of science in the West is notoriously low.[11] Western government ministers and officials sometimes suffer from the same ignorance as the general public, but feel obliged to maintain independent bodies of experts, precisely to make up for these shortcomings. One way of summarising the main claim of this chapter is that in this respect parents should imitate governments, and feel obliged to consult people who know more than they do, where such knowledge is relevant to practical deliberation and discussion.

Unfortunately, the policy decisions of governments sometimes seem to foster a false sense of expertise in parents specifically, and the public at large in general. For example, when parents are told that the choice of schools for their children should be up to them, or that they have the right to overrule and challenge teachers in school though their own education is abysmal, that may foster an illusion of being able to make the relevant judgements just in virtue of being a parent. This is just as much of an illusion as it is to think that one is expert in relation to one's child's health because one is the parent of that child. Of course, it is easier to acquire the knowledge relevant to school choice and dealing with teachers than it is to acquire the knowledge required for decisions about MMR, but the knowledge is not innate, and it does not suddenly come into being when one becomes a parent. Some parents may never acquire, and a few may be *un*able to acquire, *either* sort of knowledge.

In the MMR case expert knowledge seems highly relevant in ways that other things—strongly felt parental feelings—may not. But in other cases expert knowledge may be out of its element altogether, or may matter less because things that are not matters of expert knowledge are also relevant and weighty.

Consider the case of genetically modified (hereafter 'GM') food. There may be a majority in the UK against growing GM crops, and also against buying GM produce in the shops. Even if this consensus is based, as it seems

---

[11] It is easy to overdraw the divide between the experts and the public. Intermediaries, in the press, and in NGOs, who have the relevant expertise but are also interested in making experts accountable, can mediate between the public and experts and can equip members of the public with expert representation in the scientific community. What is more, they can aid the process of disseminating or making accessible, expertise.

to be, on very little evidence that GM crops or GM food are harmful, the fact that there would be little or no market for them if they were produced may be an argument for not developing a capacity for producing GM food products, at any rate for the time being. People could eventually be convinced that GM food was harmless, but that would not guarantee that GM food would ever be bought in sufficient quantities to make trials in the present worthwhile. Matters would stand differently if alternatives to GM food became very scarce, and GM food was easy and cheap to produce. But as things currently are in the West, the fact that GM food is unpopular may matter more than the fact that its unpopularity is due to scientific ignorance or prejudice. It is not as if people will come to harm by eating alternatives to GM food. It is not as if alternatives to GM food are scarce or unduly expensive.

In the GM food case, then, though expert knowledge is not out of its element, and though it may conflict with incorrect popular belief, other things—the fact that there is a free market in food and that people are unlikely to buy GM food; the fact that there is enough non-GM food to satisfy demand and hunger—these facts make the consequences of incorrect popular belief less than disastrous. In the MMR case, on the other hand, expert knowledge is relevant *and* the consequences of being guided by non-expert knowledge may in fact be very bad.

It might be thought that the authority of expert knowledge counts for less than the advisability of playing it safe, and that it is the principle of playing it safe that needs to be given maximum weight in the MMR and GM food cases alike. Since we don't know for sure what the effects of MMR or of growing GM food are, we should have nothing to do with either. After all, it is possible that the effects of both will be bad in ways we can't predict *and* irreversible. This argument is hard to assess, because mere possibilities on both sides cut no ice. One needs to know how *probable* it is that the dangers will be realized, or how good a *reason* there is to think that the ill effects will be irreversible. Not knowing what will happen by itself may not be enough. It is true that *sometimes* not knowing what will happen is a conclusive reason for doing nothing. It does not seem to be in the case where an effective treatment for a serious and widespread disease might well be available or in the offing, and where the dangers on the other side are hard to state convincingly. The precautionary principle, which assigns the burden of proof to innovators where the innovation might be dangerous, is harder to support the more obscure the dangers are, the less probable the occurrence of *big* dangers is, and the bigger the probabilities of big benefits to weigh in the balance against the big dangers.

The precautionary principle sometimes *seems* to be compelling in an unqualified form, because it is quietly harnessed to the assumption that the natural order is benign, so that any interventions in it or changes to it are bad or dangerous just in virtue of being interventions, other things being equal. There were signs of this in the statement quoted earlier from Healthy Child Online. The assumption that the natural order is benign may in its turn be harnessed to the principle that in a scientifically innocent state human beings would be greater beneficiaries of the natural order, because all the interventions we have already made in nature have already altered mechanisms that were present in nature to protect us. These are strongly question-begging assumptions, and we need not subscribe to them in order to subscribe to some version of the precautionary principle.

Besides, people need to be careful when they think about nature. Even if it is true in some sense that the natural order is benign, it is not necessarily going to mean that the natural order benefits the *human* members of the natural order to the extent required to prevent vast amounts of human pain and disease. Perhaps nature is impartial and seeks to benefit the life in the universe *on balance*. It's a big universe. Nature does not begin and end on this planet, still less with the species that live on it, still less with just our species. So it may be a mistake to expect the natural order to have a soft spot in its heart for this cosmically tiny speck of itself, still less a soft spot for the fraction of the speck that is human. Science may be what we need to help ourselves within the considerable limits left to us by a benign but vast and inclusive nature. My conclusion is that the precautionary principle is not as compelling as it looks, and that consensuses built upon it may be criticisable, even when it is the consensus of a large majority who want to make it an issue in a piece of democratic decision-making. In particular, an anti-GM or an anti- MMR consensus built upon the precautionary may be questionable.

This is not to say that supposed risks can simply be ignored by the political authorities, even where big numbers of affected people have no good reason to believe the risks exist. Public health measures require co-operation, and co-operation can only be got if even false public beliefs are taken seriously. 'Taken seriously' does not mean 'accepted', of course; but it does mean investigation and explanation.

Investigation is what the UK Medicines and Health Care Products Regulatory Agency (as it now is) undertook in 1998 in response to those who believed that MMR had harmed their children. Working through a solicitor's firm representing those who were bringing legal claims for damage supposedly resulting from the MMR vaccine, the Agency carefully reconstructed the medical histories of those children in whom bowel disease and autism or a more general developmental disorder could be confirmed. In many cases they found a family history of developmental disorder, difficulty in pregnancy, GP records of symptoms in the affected children before they had had the MMR vaccine; in short, a host of possible causes of symptoms *other* than the MMR vaccine. The MHRA has also attempted to rebut a 2001 article by Wakefield and Fletcher alleging that the MMR vaccine had been licensed in the UK without being sufficiently studied.[12]

Although the UK authorities do not seem to have been entirely successful in getting across to the general public the results of their studies or the efforts they have made to look into the individual cases of children, they do seem to me to have taken the right steps in response to claims about the vaccine, and they do seem to be right to carry on with a policy of licensing the MMR vaccine, even in the face of public disquiet about it. Not all public disquiet is well-founded, and sometimes the consequences of trying to assuage it are worse than forceful disagreement on the part of those in power.[13]

---

[12] For MHRA reports see: http://www.mhra.gov.uk (accessed 28 March 2006).

[13] I have been helped by discussions with, and comments on earlier drafts from, Heather Draper, Angus Dawson, Marcel Verweij, and an audience at Hull University.

7

Ethical Issues in Applying Quantitative Models for Setting Priorities in Prevention[1]

Dan W. Brock

7.1. Introduction

Several years ago I served on a committee of the Institute of Medicine (IoM) in the United States whose task was to recommend priorities for new vaccine development over the next 10 and 20 years (Institute of Medicine 2001). The project was undertaken under contract from the National Institutes of Allergy and Infectious Diseases of the National Institutes of Health. The committee's mandate required it to develop a quantitative model for determining the priorities that it would recommend. In the committee's discussion about what model to employ cost effectiveness quite naturally quickly rose to the forefront of alternatives for several reasons. First,

[1] This chapter draws on several of my previous efforts on this topic, most especially material I contributed to Institute of Medicine (2001), as well as two of my own papers (Brock 2004a, b). Others of my previous publications on these topics are referenced within the paper.

the methodology of cost-effectiveness analysis (CEA) has been extensively explored and developed, in particular for use in health policy. The US Public Health Service Panel had just completed its extensive study, *Cost-Effectiveness in Health and Medicine*, which included a variety of recommendations on technical issues in carrying out such analyses in the health context (Gold et al. 1996). Second, the normative principle underlying CEA appears to many people, especially in public health, to be almost self-evidently correct. That principle is that limited resources available for health should be used so as to maximize the health benefits for the population served. Third, unlike cost-benefit analysis (CBA), CEA does not require placing a monetary value on life which many find problematic in practice as well as morally objectionable; this is one of the reasons why CEAs are much more common in the health field than CBAs. Fourth, despite common ethical objections to CEA grounded in concerns for justice or equity, there is no consensus on many of these equity issues which could have been drawn on in order to incorporate specific positions on equity into the model. In the literature as it then existed and now exists, there is not only no widely accepted alternative quantitative model incorporating those equity considerations, but there is no such quantitative alternative, widely accepted or not. Instead, there are various ethical objections that moral philosophers, bioethicists and others have raised to the use of CEA for prioritization in the health sector, and empirical studies that elicit some of the respects in which people's priorities diverge from CEA in setting health sector priorities. But there is no comprehensive alternative quantitative model to CEA that incorporates a comprehensive account of justice or equity.

As a result of considerations like these, the IoM committee adopted CEA as the quantitative model for determining its recommendations for new vaccine development. Vaccines are of course only one preventive strategy in public health and the issues that arise in determining priorities for their development arise more broadly for other prevention initiatives in public health. This use of CEA for setting priorities in prevention programs raises two broad issues that I will explore in this chapter. What are the ethical issues that arise in applying quantitative models like CEA in setting priorities for prevention in the health sector (see Brock 2004a, b)? Should alternative quantitative models to CEA be developed that incorporate specific accounts of equity or justice (Daniels 1998)? I shall spend more time on the first question, but once we have addressed it we will be in a better position to try to answer the second. It needs to be emphasized at the outset that the first question is large and complex and I will only be able to summarize briefly here some of the main issues, many of which I and others have written about more extensively elsewhere.

7.2. Ethical and Value Assumptions in CEA

7.2.1. Valuing Benefits and Costs

CEA requires a measure of benefits and of costs in order to assess different preventive interventions for their relative cost-effectiveness, that is, for the amount of benefit they produce for a unit of cost. Costs are standardly measured in monetary terms and I will take up shortly what costs should be counted, but greater ethical controversy surrounds the measurement of benefits. The standard measure of benefits is some version of the quality adjusted life year (QALY) which encompasses the two main benefits that preventive health interventions provide for individuals—prevention of premature loss of life and of avoidable declines in health related quality of life. Thus, the QALYs from a particular preventive intervention for a particular subject of the intervention are determined by the additional years of life produced for the subject and/or the increase in the health related quality of life for the subject. In evaluating alternative health prevention efforts for the same individual, just as in evaluating alternative treatments for the same individual patient, it is relatively uncontroversial that the alternative that produces the most QALYs should be preferred; issues of equity do not arise. This simply reflects the fact that, so long as people's quality of life remains acceptable to them, they prefer to live longer and with a higher health related quality of life. (Of course, often tradeoffs between length and quality of life must be made, but the QALY measure in principle allows those tradeoffs to be made.)

Different preventive interventions, however, such as the development and use of vaccines are often aimed at different populations or different subgroups within a population, and then issues of equity do arise. Even if alternative preventive interventions are aimed at the same population they may affect different subgroups within that population differently, for example males versus females or different ethnic or racial groups, and then equity issues again can arise. This may be an especially important issue for the prioritization of different preventive interventions as opposed to therapeutic or curative interventions. Preventive interventions are often targeted at relatively homogeneous subgroups within a population whereas therapeutic interventions are typically targeted at more heterogeneous groups consisting of all those with a particular disease. There are also some equity issues that have special importance in the prioritization of preventive versus therapeutic interventions, in particular the discounting of health benefits which is discussed below.

The intervention producing the most QALYs still is plausibly considered to produce the greater overall health benefit, to have a greater positive impact on population health. Since protecting and promoting population health is often assumed to be the goal of preventive interventions and of public health more generally, this may seem to support maximizing QALYs as the standard for evaluating prevention interventions. I will argue shortly that considerations of equity or fairness properly constrain the goal, but some version of QALYs does seem to be a plausible measure of health benefits.

QALYs require a quantitative measure of health related quality of life in different medical conditions or different conditions of disability or limited function. This is typically done with a measure like the Health Utilities Index on which death is valued at zero and full health at one (Horsman et al. 2003). Various states of disability are then valued on this scale by asking individuals their preferences for being in a given state using standard gambles, time tradeoffs, visual analogue scales, or person tradeoffs. One concern about these methodologies is that they let other values influence the values assigned to health states—attitudes to risk affect standard gambles, time preferences affect time tradeoffs, and equity concerns affect person tradeoffs (Solomon & Murray 2002). A second issue is whose preferences should be used to value different health states (Menzel et al. 2002). The main controversy has been whether to use the preferences of persons who are actually in the particular health state with the disability in question or the preferences of the general population. The reason this matters is that a number of studies have shown that persons with various disabilities tend to rate them as less bad than do others who have not experienced them. One reason for this difference is simply a variety of prejudices, stereotypes, and false beliefs about life with disabilities held by much of the public. In addition, persons typically adapt to their disabilities by learning to perform functions in new ways, adapting their life plans to their disabilities, and adjusting their expectations to their functional limitations (Solomon and Murray 2002). In so doing they adopt new valuational perspectives from which they assess their health related quality of life. Neither their earlier nor their adapted valuational perspective is mistaken—the difference is the result of a change based on the individual's new circumstances, with the latter perspective reflecting the new restriction in abilities and opportunities (Brock 1995). The importance of this issue for the evaluation of prevention programs is that the higher evaluation of health related quality of life in various states of disability of persons who have the disability in question will result in less value assigned to programs that prevent such states of disability. This issue is broader than just the implications for the evaluation of prevention programs and there is no consensus in the literature on it.

7.2.2. Discount Rates

One important issue in doing a CEA of health programs of especial importance for prevention programs is whether a discount rate should be applied to benefits and costs that arise at some point in the future (Murray 1996). For many prevention programs, the costs of the program must be incurred at the time the program is carried out, while the health benefits occur at some future time. In typical examples such as vaccination programs or programs to change unhealthy behaviors, the benefits of the programs often come many years after the initial intervention. Standard practice in CEAs is to apply a discount rate, such as 3 or 5% annually, to both benefits and costs of programs evaluated (Lipscomp et al. 1996). For familiar reasons it is uncontroversial that a discount rate should be applied to monetary benefits and costs. If monetary benefits are received now instead of several years into the future, they can be invested producing a greater overall sum at that future time than if they were not received until later. If costs can be postponed without postponing or changing the benefits, then funds can be invested until costs must be paid and fewer current dollars will be needed to meet costs. Moreover, if future benefits are more uncertain than nearer benefits, which will only sometimes be the case, those benefits should be discounted for this uncertainty. And finally, if getting a health improvement sooner or postponing a health burden until later produces a greater total benefit over time, that too is a reason for preferring the earlier benefit or the later burden. But neither of these last two points requires applying a discount rate to health benefits—they are accommodated simply by an assessment of overall health benefits, discounted for uncertainty.

The ethical issue is whether a health benefit of a given size, say extending 1000 people's lives by ten years, has less social value and so should receive a lower priority merely because it occurs say 10 years in the future instead of today. To apply a discount rate to health benefits is to answer this question affirmatively. It is to hold that we should prefer a smaller health benefit now to a larger one in the future, merely because that later benefit occurs in the future rather than now. There is a large literature on discounting that there is no space to review here—I can only note without any defense that I do not believe there is a persuasive ethical justification for discounting health benefits, although this issue remains highly controversial (Lazaro 2002).

I would reiterate the importance of this point for prioritization of prevention programs. Such programs typically accrue their health benefits some significant time into the future, and so applying a discount rate to their benefits will systematically disadvantage them in comparison with most acute care programs whose benefits usually accrue relatively immediately; this disadvantaging is despite equal or greater health benefits from the prevention programs. And even within prioritization among different prevention programs, applying a discount rate to health benefits can result in giving higher priority to programs that produce lesser aggregate health benefits than alternative programs, merely because the lesser benefits come sooner.

7.2.3. Indirect and Non-Health Benefits and Costs

Another issue in the calculation of the benefits and costs of prevention and other health programs concerns what benefits and costs should be counted (Brock 2003a). It is uncontroversial that the direct health benefits to program recipients in preserving or prolonging life and in protecting or improving health related quality of life should count. Likewise, it is uncontroversial that direct program costs such as equipment and supplies, medical personnel time, and so forth should count. But many health programs have indirect and/or non health benefits and costs that can be sufficiently large to swamp their direct benefits and costs. For example, successful substance abuse prevention programs not only produce health benefits for participants, but produce large indirect benefits such as reducing costs of lost work time to employers, reducing crime, reducing burdens to family members, and so forth. Should this fact increase such programs' priority? On the one hand these are real costs of substance abuse, even if not health costs, and real benefits of a successful prevention effort. On the other hand, to do so values preventing these patients potential illnesses more highly than those with otherwise comparable health needs without these indirect benefits because meeting their needs has indirect benefits to others. This sets priorities on the basis of people's social value to others, as opposed to the urgency of their health needs. Counting indirect effects like lost wages would discriminate against prevention programs for conditions that typically strike during people's non-working years—childhood and old age—and would discriminate against low wage workers with less than average lost wages.

There are other examples where doing a CEA taking account of all costs and benefits, whether direct or indirect and whether health or non-health, of a preventive intervention is problematic on ethical grounds. It has often been noted that preventing smoking may not be cost-effective despite smoking's large health costs because people often die of smoking related diseases about the time of retirement and their death forestalls public pension costs as well as future health costs. From the perspective of a government funding pension and health programs, these are real effects on its public accounts. Yet few would take these costs as a reason to give lower priority to smoking prevention (Menzel 1990, Ch 4). This illustrates that on both the benefits and costs side of a CEA some consequences of prevention programs may have to be ignored on ethical grounds if we are to give equal moral concern to people's health care needs.

7.2.4. Age Weighting

Standard practice in CEA is to assign equal size health benefits the same value, whatever the age of their recipients. However, in its work on summary measures of population health and on CEAs of various health interventions, the WHO assigned different value to health benefits depending on the age of the recipients of the benefits (Murray 1994). In particular, it assigned lesser value to benefits for young children and the elderly, and greater value to benefits for adults in their productive working years, The rationale for this was that young children and the elderly typically were economically, socially, and psychologically dependent on working age adults. This was an ethically problematic justification for their age weighting because it assigned greater value to health benefits for working age adults because of their greater instrumental social value to others. It would seemingly violate giving equal moral weight to the equal health needs of individuals and would have other implications in conflict with equity, such as giving greater value to the health needs of the more productive members of society.

There are other justifications for some age-weighting, however, that may be justified on grounds of fairness, at least for life extending health benefits. This justification would assign greater moral or social value to prevention programs for life-threatening conditions, the younger the individuals whose lives would otherwise be threatened without those programs. While the position can be specified in various ways, the basic idea is that the younger an individual is who loses her life when that loss might have been prevented, the greater the unfairness. Fairness requires, on this view, that so far as possible each individual have the life years necessary for a normal lifespan, or what Alan Williams has called a 'fair innings' (Williams 1997). Fairness in this view requires favoring younger persons over older persons in distributing additional life years through prevention programs, that is, favoring those who will have had less of the good of life years if they do receive the prevention program that would benefit them. Many will charge that favoring younger over older persons for life-extending prevention programs amounts to unjust age discrimination, and it is certainly true that doing so would be controversial. But doing so is unlike other forms of discrimination, such as that against women or particular racial or ethnic groups (Daniels 1988). While individuals remain a member of only one sex or racial or ethnic group, each individual can expect to pass through different stages of a normal lifespan. Favoring the young over the old treats every individual or group equally when they are at the same age, although individuals will reach a particular age at different times. Since the justification suggested above for doing so is specifically grounded in fairness, merely charging age discrimination is inadequate without rebutting that argument from fairness.

7.3. Ethical Issues in the Use of CEA

The issues discussed briefly above concern ethical assumptions typical in most CEAs, and whether those assumptions are justified. Once a CEA has been done, there are additional issues raised for its use for prioritization of prevention programs by the fact that it ignores several issues of equity, three of the most important of which are discussed below.

7.3.1. The Aggregation Problem

What has come to be called the aggregation problem concerns whether only the overall aggregate benefits and costs of alternative health programs should be compared for the purposes of prioritization? Standard practice in CEA, as well as in its philosophical foundations of utilitarianism or consequentialism, is to prioritize only on the basis of overall aggregate benefits and costs. This also fits with the goal of seeking to maximize a population's health. Placing no limits on aggregation in this way, however, ignores how benefits and costs of prevention programs are distributed to different individuals or groups.

Perhaps the most common version of the aggregation problem concerns the comparison of small benefits to many individuals with large benefits to a much smaller number of individuals. The best known illustration of the problem arose when the state of Oregon set out to revise its Medicaid program about 15 years ago (Garland 1992). Initially using what was essentially a CE standard, it ranked over 700 treatment/condition pairs, that is, treatments provided to patients in specific conditions. In its initial list, capping teeth was ranked just above appendectomies for acute appendicitis, despite the fact that the latter condition is life threatening. While there were various technical objections to Oregon's methodology and their use of it, including in this instance its cost estimates for the procedures, this is the kind of result that can be expected with CEA. Oregon estimated that it could treat over 100 patients in need of tooth capping for the cost of treating one patient in need of an appendectomy, and that the aggregate benefit of treating those 100+ patients exceeded that of treating the one patient for acute appendicitis. This result was widely rejected and led the Oregon Health Services Commission to revise its prioritization methodology. It rejected a CE standard in place of what was largely a relative benefit standard, with cost differences largely ignored except as tie breakers for equally effective interventions. Oregon's experience reflected that most people's intuitive prioritization rankings are based on a one-to-one comparison of different treatments or conditions prevented, in which case an appendectomy is clearly of higher priority than tooth capping.

The aggregation problem can arise not only from differences in the costs of preventing a health problem in each affected individual, but also from differences in the incidence of different diseases in a population and this is probably its most common form in an area of prevention programs like development and use of vaccines. Here are examples in the area of vaccines we cited in the

IoM report. Very serious but relatively uncommon diseases like meningitis or tetanus may have to be compared with much less serious but much more common diseases like chicken pox, mononucleosis (Epstein-Barr virus) or diarrhea (caused by rotavirus and other infectious agents). The latter may create an overall greater disease burden, while the former create a much greater disease burden for each individual who contracts them. CEA will often give higher priority to preventing the high-incidence/low-individual−burden disease than to preventing the low-incidence/high-individual−burden disease.

Do people's intuitive priorities based on one-to-one comparisons of different diseases to be prevented simply represent a mistaken failure to take account of differences in cost or incidence? In fact there may be ethical reasons behind this common ignoring, or at least downplaying, of cost or incidence differences in common thinking about priorities. In some empirical studies, many individuals express the view that people should not have a lower priority for treatment (and by extension prevention) simply because their diseases are more expensive to treat (or prevent) (Nord et al. 1995). Likewise, people should not have a lower priority in the development of treatments or prevention efforts simply because their diseases have a much lower incidence in the population than competing priorities; so-called orphan drug development programs may reflect this view. A somewhat different way of defending ignoring differences in cost or incidence can be found in contractualist and some other non-consequentialist moral theories (Scanlon 1998). The idea is that individuals should confront other individuals, not aggregates of individuals, in competitions for scarce resources and we should give priority to the individuals with the strongest or most urgent claims or needs. Those individuals with the most urgent needs will have the greatest complaints if their needs are not met, and we should attempt to minimize the complaints of those who have the greatest or strongest complaint.

The complexity of this issue is that while many people are not prepared to accept the unlimited aggregation of CEA and utilitarianism, they are also not prepared to reject all aggregation. The task then is to delineate when, and for what reasons, aggregation is ethically acceptable and when it is not.

7.3.2. Priority to the Worst Off

It is a commonplace that justice requires special concern for the worst off. This is reflected in the principles of prominent theories of justice, such as

John Rawls' Difference Principle, in aphorisms like 'you can tell the justice of a society by how it treats its least well off members,' and within many religious traditions by their special concern for the poor (Rawls 1971). In the context of prioritization of public health prevention programs, there are three principal question regarding this priority: Why give priority to the worst off? Who are the worst off? How much priority should the worst off receive? The potential answers to the first question are various and cannot be explored here (Brock 2002). It is, however, important to distinguish priority to the worse off from a concern for equality. Of course, raising the position of the worse off will often reduce inequality as well, but the two concerns are nevertheless fundamentally different. What has been called Prioritarianism holds that it is morally more important to benefit people the worse off those people are. Prioritarians are concerned with the absolute position of the worse off (Parfit 1991). A concern for equality, on the other hand, is concerned with people's position relative to others in some respect and that they be equal in that respect. Many have rejected the egalitarian position in favor of Prioritarianism because the former is subject to the leveling down objection (Parfit 1991). It is possible to increase equality not by bringing up the position of the worse off, but by bringing down the position of the better off, even if doing so in no way benefits the worse off; many find this objection against egalitarianism in outcomes decisive.

Let us assume then, what I have not argued for here, that a justification grounded in justice or fairness, can be found for giving priority to the worse off. But who are the worse off in the context of prioritization of prevention programs? They might be those who are globally or overall worse off, such as the poor, or those with worse health, that is, the sickest; these will often, but not always, be the same individuals or groups. Like the other issues taken up in this chapter, this one too cannot be explored fully here. If we take the global perspective, then we could be committed to giving priority to prevention programs directed at the poor for substantially less serious conditions than to those faced by better off classes. If we give priority to those with worse health, does that mean, in the case of prevention programs, worse health before the prevention program is initiated, or those whose health would be worse if the prevention program is not initiated. These will not always be the same, but either interpretation would imply that sometimes we should sacrifice some aggregate health benefits for the sake of preventing health losses to those with worse health.

Finally, even if some priority should be given to prevention programs for the poor or those with worse health, the question remains how much priority. Giving them absolute priority is implausible because it could result in foregoing unlimited benefits from prevention programs not serving the worst off in order to secure minimal benefits to the worse off; this has been called the 'bottomless pit' problem. But there seems no unique principled solution to how much priority to give to prevention programs, or for that matter treatment programs, serving the worse off. Like most of the other equity issues addressed in this chapter, this too is an issue on which reasonable people disagree, even within one society or country much less across different societies or countries. I will take up the implications of this disagreement for quantitative models, as well as for health policy decision making, later in this chapter.

7.3.3. Fair Chances versus Best Outcomes

CEA is the analytic measure for determining which alternative use of resources will produce the best outcome in health benefits. If we always choose the resource use that produces the best outcome then those who would be served by a less than best alternative resource use will have no chance of having their needs met when resource scarcity does not permit funding both alternatives. Always preferring the alternative that produces best outcomes will be most ethically problematic when the differences between the cost effectiveness of alternative resource uses is small but the difference in outcomes for individuals is very large depending on which alternative is funded, in the extreme case the difference between life and death.

The thesis that resources should be targeted to preventive interventions in which they will do the most good entails a higher priority to those who can be helped cheaply, whether in prevention versus prevention or prevention versus therapeutic comparisons. This in turn implies that some patients will lose out simply because their needs are more expensive to meet. Consider, for example, two otherwise similar prevention programs that would serve the same number of persons and produce comparable overall benefits, but one of which is more expensive because it would serve a rural instead of an urban population. The program serving the urban population is more cost-effective, but those in the rural area could argue that it is unfair to give them no chance to have their needs met merely because meeting them is somewhat more expensive. Limited surveys indicate a sharp difference between health professionals, who tend to favor the cost-effective alternative, and the general public, who tend to favor giving all in need a chance at needed treatment or prevention, in their responses to this conflict. This division of opinion goes to the heart of CEA, which is precisely a guide to identifying the route to the best outcomes that can be hoped for with existing resources. It creates a dilemma for those health professionals who maintain that health policy should be based on values most frequently endorsed by the population affected.

The conflict between fair chances and best outcomes arises not only from differences in the costs of treating otherwise similar groups of patients, but also when one group of patients will receive somewhat greater benefits than another at the same cost. The appeal of a fair-chances solution is greater where the difference in cost-effectiveness between the two programs is relatively small relative to the potential gain or loss to each affected individual. Consider two prevention programs that would serve different, but equal size, populations at equal cost. Program A will produce 5000 QALYs while B will produce 4500 QALYs, and the impact on the health of life on each patient served is very large. Patients who would be served by B could complain that it is not fair that all the resources go to A and none to B when they have nearly as pressing health risks and would be benefited by prevention nearly as much as the individuals served by A. If all cannot receive prevention efforts, they might go on to argue, they deserve a fair chance to have their needs met rather than having no chance for prevention efforts because serving them would produce slightly less overall benefit than serving the individuals in A. The small difference in benefits produced for the two groups, they argue, is too small to justify the very great difference in how the two groups are treated—for example, individuals served by A avoid a very serious long term disability and individuals who would be served by B suffer an only slightly less serious disability. Or it might be a matter of life and death, and individuals in A have a slightly higher life expectancy than those in B. Note that there is no challenge to the fact that more good or a better outcome is produced by funding program A rather than B, only that that the additional good is insufficient to justify morally the very great difference in the way the two groups of patients are treated.

Preferring the most cost-effective program can also seem unfair because it compounds existing unfair inequalities. For example, screening slum dwelling black men for hypertension targets the group with the highest incidence and greatest risk of premature death, but it is more cost-effective to target well-to-do suburban white men, since they have more ordered lives, comply better, have personal doctors and the means to obtain medical services, are more educated and more likely to modify their lifestyles wisely, etc. But if the poor blacks are not screened for this reason, it only compounds their existing unjust deprivation, and of course is also in conflict with giving priority to the worst off.

If those who need a less cost-effective program deserve a fair chance to have their needs met, what would be a fair chance? There is controversy about this. Some argue that a fair chance is an equal chance and so some random method of selecting which program to fund should be used. Others have suggested proportional chances or a weighted lottery in which the chance of each program being selected is proportional to the amount of health benefit each would produce; this would be a way of balancing fair chances against best outcomes. Or some resources might go to each program if that is possible, thereby benefiting some patients in each group. However fair chances is interpreted, it can be argued that at the macro level of allocation where resources for prevention programs are usually divisible, unlike for example a scarce life saving organ needed by two potential transplant recipients, some resources should be devoted to the different alternative programs, at least if their relative benefits are not strikingly dissimilar, instead of all going to the most cost effective programs.

7.3.4. The Equity Considerations—Within or Outside of the Quantitative Model?

I have delineated briefly above several of the ethical issues that are raised by the most common quantitative analysis, CEA, employed for health resource prioritization generally, and for prevention programs in particular. In general, CEA ignores concerns for equity or justice and contains several ethically controversial assumptions. Should we then seek to develop an alternative quantitative methodology that incorporates these ethical concerns and/or alternative ethical assumptions (Nord et al. 1999)? This is a complex issue on which there are conflicting considerations and no consensus. Some researchers have done empirical studies using the person tradeoff methodology to determine how much individuals are prepared to sacrifice in aggregate health benefits in order, for example, to ensure that the sickest receive treatment;

as noted above, this is one interpretation of the equity concern to give some special priority to the worse off (Nord 1993). To date, such studies have been limited in several respects. They have generally only involved relatively small and often nonrepresentative respondents, and the validity and stability of the results are not well established. Moreover, similar empirical work has not been done on some of the other equity issues discussed above. So at the present time more research is needed before it would be possible to incorporate the full range of equity concerns in a quantitative methodology for prioritization. However, this might still be a longer term goal. A quantitative approach can have a powerful attraction and impact in many health policy contexts and it could be argued that unless there is a quantitative alternative to CEA that incorporates equity considerations, the utilitarian maximization approach of CEA will inevitably have a disproportionate influence and equity considerations will not get proper attention and weight.

Despite these considerations, there remain serious difficulties with pursuing the strategy of quantifying considerations of equity as an alternative to CEA (Daniels 1998). Some have argued that it is desirable to leave CEA as a measure only of the relative goodness or health benefits produced by alternative preventive strategies, with equity or fairness concerns considered separately. However, this pure separation is rarely achieved in practice; for example, diseases that attack the economically productive middle and upper classes are rarely given higher priority for that reason in a CEA than those that attack the poor. Nevertheless, it is possible to keep most equity or fairness considerations separate from a CEA which would remain, at least largely, a measure of goodness. This has the advantage of making clearer how much by way of aggregate goodness or health benefits would be sacrificed in order to meet various equity concerns.

A deeper difficulty with the goal of incorporating various equity concerns within a quantitative measure analogous to CEA is that there is no consensus on many of the equity issues in question, either among the general public or within work in moral philosophy and health policy. For example, there is no consensus about whether additional life years should be given greater social value, the younger their recipient, as the fair innings argument would imply, or when or how much we should depart from CEAs implications in order to give people a fair chance to have their needs met. Who, if anyone, should have special priority, and how much, in order to give special priority to the worst off? Indeed, virtually all of the equity concerns raised above are controversial, and yet a quantitative measure that incorporates them requires taking precise positions on each of them. If, for example, as some studies show a significant proportion of the population would favor maximizing health benefits, while another significant proportion would favor substantial priority to the sickest, what position should we incorporate into the quantitative standard? If we split the difference, or compromise between their conflicting positions, we may end with a position that neither group supports.

If, despite these difficulties, quantitative measures that incorporate equity considerations are pursued then one alternative to at least partially deal with the ethical controversies about the equity issues is to employ sensitivity analyses for different positions on those issues. For example, on the issue of whether to apply discount rates to health benefits in CEAs the World Health Organization has in some of its work run sensitivity analyses comparing results with and without a discount rate applied to health benefits. In principle this would be possible for other equity issues as well, although the relevant alternative positions to test for are not as well defined with many of the other equity concerns and the array of alternative results would increase markedly as the number of issues and alternative positions on which sensitivity analyses are run increases.

The other principal alternative for taking account of equity considerations is to leave the quantitative measure at least largely a measure of the cost-effectiveness for overall goodness or health benefits and then to rely on the political process or policy maker to take account of the additional equity issues. Too often, a CEA for some health policy choice is simply accompanied by an admonition to the policy maker that the CEA does not take account of concerns for equity and so the policy maker should do so, but with little if any guidance about what those specific concerns are or how the policy maker might address them. In such circumstances it should be no surprise that the equity concerns are given no or inadequate consideration. Instead, what policy makers require is guidance on what specific equity concerns are raised by the policy choice in question and what are plausible alternative positions on them, as well as the reasons in support of those alternatives.

In practice, it will often be health policy makers who make use of quantitative methodologies like CEA for prioritizing alternative preventive strategies and programs. The absence of consensus about most of the equity issues discussed above implies that to ensure the fairness of the standards used by policy makers for prioritization we may have to rely on fair procedures for making those prioritization choices. It is beyond the scope of this chapter to give a full account of fair procedures for prioritization of prevention programs. Among other things, the details of such procedures will vary depending on the specific context in which such decisions are made—for example, at the international level by an organization like WHO, at the country level in a health ministry, at a regional level by regional health authorities, within a managed care plan or health maintenance organization, and so forth. But there is fairly widespread agreement that for procedures to be fair and to confer legitimacy on the specific priorities determined by them, at least the following conditions advanced by Norman Daniels should be met:

1. *Publicity Condition*: The process must be transparent and involve publicly available rationales for the priorities that are set;

2. *Relevance Condition*: Stakeholders affected by these decisions must agree that the rationales rest on reasons, principles and evidence they view as relevant to making fair decisions about priorities; community and stakeholder participation and voice must vary in an appropriate way with institutional context;

3. *Revisability and Appeals Condition*: The process allows for revisiting and revising decisions in light of new evidence and arguments, and allows for an appeals process that protects those who have legitimate reasons for being an exception to policies adopted.

4. *Enforcement or Regulation Condition*: There is a mechanism in place that assures the previous three conditions are met.

(Daniels 2004)

A procedure that meets these conditions at least ensures individuals with different interests and different conceptions of equity that their interests and views have been given fair consideration in the prioritization process, even if some are favored and some disfavored.

7.4. Conclusion

CEA is the dominant quantitative methodology used in the health sector for prioritizing different prevention programs, but it is widely accepted that it ignores concerns about equity. We have reviewed briefly some of the principal issues of equity raised by CEA. Public health officials and others engaged in prioritizing prevention programs should not simply choose the most cost-effective programs, but instead should balance concern for cost-effectiveness with the various concerns about equity discussed above. Whether quantitative methodologies can or should be developed that incorporate positions on the various equity issues is controversial and we have discussed some of the difficulties and objections to attempting to do so.

8

Reasonable Limits to Public Health Demands[1]

Mariëtte van den Hoven

8.1. Introduction

With an increasing frequency, individuals in Western countries are confronted with preventive programmes. These activities vary from offers of
general screening and immunisation programmes to specific lifestyle and
nutritional recommendations; for example, you can be tested for choles-
terol while shopping in the supermarket, buy step-o-meters to measure
your physical activity, or you can obtain preconception information about
possible genetic risks when deciding to have children.

In the jungle of public health we often simply assume that *each* individual
will benefit from all these recommendations and offers. However, this is
not true. Rose once pointed to the paradoxical situation that 'a preventive
measure that brings large benefits to the community can afford little to
each participating individual' (Rose 1992). After all, public health is first and

[1] I am very much indebted to discussions with my colleagues and supervisors, Marcel Verweij
and Robert Heeger. While completing my thesis, and developing my arguments I also greatly
benefited from discussions with participants at the symposium on Public Health and Ethical
Theory, Utrecht University, May 2002 and at the workshop of the Society of Applied Philosophy,
'Public Health, Ethical Theory and Public Goods' in Gonville and Caius College, Cambridge, July
2004.

foremost a collective action taken by society to stimulate the health of the entire population. The effects of these collective actions are mainly measured statistically: non-smoking campaigns aim to reduce the number of people smoking in a population, immunisation programmes try to influence the prevalence of infectious diseases, breast cancer screening aims to reduce the number of cases of breast cancer. However, these collective aims can often only be established when a majority will comply with the screening offers and preventive actions: herd immunity cannot be obtained when a large population rejects vaccination, and screening programmes would be unsuccessful if only a small number would comply with the offer of participation.

The compliance of individuals is often presumed. It is expected that individuals will be motivated to participate because it is somehow in their individual interests to do so. There is no guarantee, however, that all preventive measures will be as effective as one may think: for example, many people choose to ignore advice about the risk of smoking.

Non-compliance and a lack of motivation to act upon health care recommendations are much discussed issues, and we frequently encounter explanations varying from a lack of competence to decide to stop smoking to a different priority that people give to the value of health and other values (like living a satisfactory life). My focus will be on one particular type of explanation that has been neglected in such discussions so far. I will argue that some requests can be held to be *unreasonable* from an agent's perspective and that this may explain non-compliance with preventive activities.

Why would the reasonableness of a demand be a relevant consideration with respect to public health measures? I will argue that it matters greatly what is expected from an individual in relation to their contribution to the overall good that public health measures aim to achieve. Some 'demands' in public health can either outweigh what one is willing to contribute, or can differ so greatly from one's current view on life that one is not willing to make the effort. Consider the case where you are expected to change your lifestyle radically in order to reduce the chance of becoming ill in the future. It can be hard for people to live up to standards that involve changing one's habits, diet, lifestyle and possibly even one's living environment. I will argue that the considerations of the person's perspective matter greatly and should be given more weight in our deliberations about public health programmes, especially when they concern a claim about the need for *reasonable* demands.

Consider an extreme example of what has proven to be extremely burdensome on agents. China has had a one-child policy since the early 1980s, encouraging people to have only one child, in order to control the enormous problems due to overpopulation. A reduction in the number of newborn children would benefit the economy and improve the health and wealth of the whole population. However, this policy may be considered an extreme measure, from an agent's perspective, likely to be burdensome and unreasonable. After all, this policy has high impact on the personal choices and lives of agents, and was enforced by a system of reward and punishment: you are rewarded with many extras if you complied with the policy and punished if you gave birth to more children.[2] This one-child policy is commonly viewed as too burdensome on agents, and as an unreasonable measure to control problems of overpopulation. In other words, when deliberating about what policies will be acceptable as a means to improve our public health, many of us would reject such extreme measures and respect some limits to what we can expect of agents. In this chapter I will argue that this notion of reasonableness and the idea that we have to respect limits to what we can impose on agents is highly relevant for public health ethics. This issue touches upon an ongoing debate in moral philosophy focusing on the possible over-burdening of agents. This has become known as the 'demandingness debate'.

8.2. Limits to Demands on Agents

The thought that some demands can be unreasonable to agents rests upon a widespread and commonly held belief that we cannot expect agents to comply with just any request. The one-child policy is intuitively rejected, because it jeopardizes an agent's free choice to procreate. We also reject the idea of donating our whole salary to charity, because it would deny agents the ability to live their own lives. However, it is one thing to have these ideas in common with others, but quite another to be justified in holding them, as, of course, we can see that most moral agents will also recognize some duties to alleviate world poverty as well as feeling some inclination to improve the public health. It is also commonly held that we have a moral duty to give aid when this will

---

[2] Notice that in China, this policy was enforced not by law, but more subtly, through a system of incentives and penalties that together encouraged people to have only one child.

be at little cost to ourselves. This is expressed in Singer's famous *Life Saving Analogy*, in which he argues that agents have a moral obligation to save the life of a child drowning in a pond when this will only cost you a wet suit (Singer 1972).

The idea, therefore, that some requests can be unreasonable does not refer to the idea that we should deny all moral responsibilities and duties, but instead that we should honour some limits to the sacrifices we can expect from agents. This is the basic idea lying behind what has become known as the demandingness debate. The debate was originally stimulated by some critical comments that Bernard Williams and others have made in relation to act-utilitarian theories. Williams suggests that a commitment to act-utilitarianism results in alienation, because it is unreasonable to expect agents to give equal weight to concerns for one's loved ones and those of a stranger (Williams 1981), or to expect agents to distance themselves from their personal interests, plans and commitments (Williams 1973). Some projects and plans matter greatly to us, because they are part of our identity. It would therefore jeopardize our integrity if we would be required to forego our own interests, in order to achieve some greater impartial good. These and other critical comments were the starting point to deliberations about whether ethical theories should respect some boundaries to the costs that can be legitimately imposed on agents.

However, this view is not undisputed. Some philosophers argue that overdemandingness is not an issue that challenges *ethical theories*. They point out that an ethical theory is primarily focused upon establishing what our ideal moral responsibilities would look like, not whether agents are capable of living up to these responsibilities in practice. They can also refer to the fact that we live in a non-ideal world, in which great misery exists. Making this world a better place may possibly involve great sacrifices from agents. Therefore, every attempt to claim that our responsibilities must be limited can be criticised. Some even go as far as to hold the view that our commonsense beliefs about reasonable demands on agents are nothing but a cover up for laziness or a defence of our convenient bourgeois morality (Murphy 2000: 15).

However, such a view is rejected from the 'commonsense' moral perspective. Commonsense moralists claim that the sacrifices that are expected from agents should be taken into account and that 'cost to the agent' is a relevant moral consideration. In what has become known as the *debate on the limits of morality* (Kagan 1989), the commonsense view offers four different arguments that such demands can be too costly, hence unreasonable to agents. Let me briefly address these arguments here.[3] First, it is argued that some of these limits are obvious: one cannot expect agents to go against a moral principle, because one cannot at the same time embrace rules against killing and harming others as well as be expected to breach them when an opportunity occurs. Other reasons also support the view that we should respect limits to the cost we can impose on agents.

Second, it is considered unreasonable if moral obligations impose huge sacrifices of time, money and effort on agents, because such demands can prevent us from leading our own lives and pursuing our own interests. Being able to lead one's own life is important to people, not only because we value freedom of choice and privacy, but also because being able to live a life of one's own is important for our identity, authenticity and integrity (Williams 1981). The one-child policy in China certainly jeopardizes the freedom of choice of individuals. We can imagine, however, that other stringent preventive measures may require someone to radically change his lifestyle and possibly even move to a different, healthier environment. This may also be highly burdensome to agents.

Third, it is burdensome to agents if they are forced to give equal consideration to strangers and their loved ones, or are required to forego commitments that derive from the latter relations in order to benefit some greater good. Williams, famously, expresses this using the phrase that for many agents it will be 'one thought too many' if someone is really expected to explain why he wants to favour his partial attitude to his wife and not benefit some stranger instead.[4] For many agents, it goes without saying that one can give priority to one's loved ones, without feeling parochial or partial. Instead, we consider it a good thing that parents care for their children and that partners, colleagues and friends spend quality time with one another.

For example, we can imagine that when the bird flu spreads among people and not enough vaccines are available to immunise people, it will be very hard for those agents responsible for the distribution of vaccines that their loved ones should be excluded from immunisation, even if there might be good reasons to follow some impartial standard. In less extreme situations, one cannot expect agents to leave their sick parents or children in order to

---

[3] I provide much more discussion of these arguments elsewhere (van den Hoven 2006).
[4] Williams (1981) borrows this example from Fried (1970).

care for a sick stranger. It is simply more obvious to care first for one's loved ones, and too burdensome to expect equal weight to be given to a stranger.

Fourth, if agents are continuously confronted with endless responsibilities and requests, this can frustrate agents and result in them becoming less interested in their moral responsibilities. If what one does seems like 'but a drop in the ocean', or if agents are completely overloaded because they are never allowed any relaxation time, this can be burdensome on agents and may no longer be considered reasonable. Consider a health-care professional, who has the general obligation to stimulate the health of her patients, but increasing knowledge about risk factors and health compromising factors has broadened her working field from care and cure to prevention as well. The many ways preventive measures can be taken—varying from actions to prevent immobility and loneliness among the elderly, give them extra nutrition, immunise them, and so on and so on, makes it an impossible job to live up to in relation to all recommendations. Somehow we have to accept that we must choose between all these measures and not expect health care professionals to live up to impossible expectations.

Based on these four arguments, commonsense morality defends the view that a possible overload to agents should be taken seriously. It urges us to accept a broad view as to what can be costly to agents, contrary to traditional debates in which demandingness is mainly conceived as the negative effects on an agent's well-being. On this view, we cannot accept that the frustrating effects or the possibility that one should do a moral wrong to another, only effects an agent's well-being. The effects of these actions are more fundamental and have consequences for one's moral agency and one's integrity. Therefore commonsense morality lays a claim on the demandingness debate that the cost to the agent should (1) be accepted as a morally relevant consideration, and, that it is (2) broader than the effects on an agent's well-being only. It is not strange that the demandingness debate so far has mainly focused on the effects on an agent's well-being, because the debate started as a critique of consequentialist theories, especially act-utilitarian views. It is wrong, however to think that only consequentialist theories can be highly demanding on agents, or that other ethical theoretical perspective will not be demanding in an equal way. The commonsense claim in the demandingness debate can therefore find support by involving other ethical perspectives in our analysis. I will show how in different ethical theories another focus on what can count as 'cost to the agent' appears that supports the four arguments that I presented above. This can best be done with the help of a case study.

8.3. Influenza Vaccination in Nursing Homes

Influenza immunisation is a fascinating example of public health activity. For healthy adults, influenza is usually not a serious illness, but for the elderly, serious effects and even (premature) death can occur.[5] Therefore the immunisation of the elderly is strongly recommended. In nursing homes, residents are usually elderly and in fragile health; hence in many places all residents are offered immunisation annually. However, residents are not optimally protected by immunisation, because they do not respond as well to immunisation as healthy people do. A better means to guarantee optimal protection seems therefore to strive at collective protection, such as the creation of herd immunity, in order to lower the chance that an outbreak of influenza will occur in a nursing home. This collective protection will involve not only the immunisation of all residents, but also of those persons who are in close contact with residents as well. Hence health care professionals are also encouraged to receive vaccination. We can certainly expect positive effects from their immunisation, since recent reports show correlations between the immunisation among staff and the incidence of influenza in nursing homes, and it is plausible that the staff are a key vector in spreading the virus (Coles et al. 1992; Carman et al. 2000). It, therefore, may seem a reasonable expectation that health care workers are immunised. However, it depends greatly on the way such expectations are implemented in practice, because there is a significant difference between kindly asking them to consider immunisation and simply mandating it. The latter, I will argue, is too demanding. It might be argued that it is an unreasonable request, even if we consider some reasons that speak in favour of special responsibilities of health care workers to prevent influenza illness. I will present two arguments that will support the view that health care workers should be prepared to make an extra effort for the protection of the health of residents. I will then present some considerations that argue for the opposite. I will conclude that such a request can still be seen to be too demanding.

---

[5] I ignore the special case of influenza pandemics here.

8.3.1. Responsibilities Towards a Collective and as a Professional

It is interesting that many nursing homes try to establish herd immunity, because herd immunity can be conceived as a collective aim (Verweij and van den Hoven 2005). We could therefore argue that either health care professionals are obligated because they are part of the collective (that is, the herd to be protected) or they have a special relationship to the collective due to their professional status (van den Hoven and Verweij 2003). I will address both arguments and show that this supports the view that we can expect health care workers to be prepared to put some extra effort into the prevention of influenza illness within the institutions where they work.

One can have different types of responsibilities as a member of a collective, depending on the characteristics of the collective we are talking about. Postema, for example, argues that we have to separate congruent and converging interests from the interests we have in the existence of a collective good. He argues that these three interests can lead to different types of responsibilities (Postema 1987).

Congruent interests are a collection of specific interests of the same kind that are held by a large and indefinite number of private individuals. *These collective interests are not based on the striving for the same goal, but on distinct objectives that have the same X-ish kind.* The danger of a terrorist attack can be considered as a good example of a congruent interest, because many people have the same interest in being saved and not being harmed by terrorists, while it is impossible to point out who exactly will actually be affected when an attack occurs, because such an attack can be carried out by a bomb in the central station, an attack during a rock concert and so on. No one can predict who will be harmed, but all share the same interest in preventing its occurrence.

With respect to our case, we can say that within nursing homes the collective protection against influenza illness can at least be based on a congruent interest, because amongst residents and staff there are certain, non-identifiable individuals that will have a direct interest in protection against the flu, as all are part of the larger group. This supports the idea that we should collectively strive at herd immunity.

One has a *convergent interest* in a collective if all the members within that community share an interest with regard to a specific thing or event. In other words, we have overlapping interests that surpass the individual perspective.

Peace, to ward off economic depressions or health threatening epidemics are considered as typical examples of convergent interests. Convergent interests are public in a stronger sense than the congruent interests, because for this type of interest, all individuals actually have an interest in the particular goal motivating action, while congruent interests involve a number of individuals that cannot be specified within the collective; it could be any one of us.

When an outbreak of influenza would occur, the whole nursing home would suffer as a result. Residents who are ill will need extra care, there would be a shortage of staff due to absenteeism, and this will put the staff's caring activities under high pressure. Hence, daily routine and community life within a nursing home could suffer greatly from an influenza epidemic. We could therefore argue that health care workers do not only have a congruent, but also a convergent interest in the prevention of influenza illness. After all, it will have direct consequences for them if an outbreak occurred.

Postema considers a third category, which supplies the strongest type of a collective interest. If we share a collective good as members of a collective, we view something as 'ours' and consider some ideal or good to *express a view of who and what we are*. This implies that the value of a collective good is independent of the actual interests of agents; it is a genuine common value. Community membership and public symbols are typical collective goods. It is hard to see why the prevention of influenza immunisation would be such a collective good. Only if within an institution the prevention of epidemics and a particular way of life would be considered as an ideal, could one argue that prevention of influenza could be conceived as some sort of collective good. I do not think that such ideals are very common within such institutions.

Based on the idea that health care professionals can at least recognize a congruent and a convergent interest in preventing influenza outbreaks, we can argue that a specific appeal can be made to them. We can expect that they are more willing to contribute to a collective action, because either those we cannot identify will greatly benefit, or all have a direct interest in the prevention of outbreaks. Thus, based on the fact that health care professionals are members of the collective, they can be appointed a special responsibility to prevent influenza.

In a second way, health care professionals can be ascribed a special responsibility, which is in their role as a *professional health care worker*. As health care professional the health and well-being of one's patients is a primary value and specific responsibilities can be assigned to professionals to support this value. We can, for example, expect health care professionals to have the skills and knowledge to provide optimal care. This involves more than knowledge about diseases and how to cure a patient; we can also expect them to take sufficient hygienic measures, like wearing a uniform and washing their hands after treating a patient, in order to prevent infections. From this perspective, it seems reasonable to expect health care workers to be at least aware of the dangers of influenza illness among residents and about health compromising factors. If, as studies show, health care professionals are most likely to spread the virus through the organisation, this suggests that they have to take extra preventive measures. Thus the least that can be expected is that they stay home when feeling ill. Accepting immunisation will be a far more effective means of avoiding spreading viruses within the nursing home and so we might expect them to accept immunisation as well.

8.3.2. Cost of Immunization to Health Care Professionals

I provided two reasons why we can expect health care professionals to put some extra effort into the prevention of influenza illness in nursing homes. In this section I will present some considerations that suggest that such extra efforts, when imposed or demanded from the staff, may be unreasonable and burdensome.

Though one can safely assume that health care workers will have an obligation to prevent infection, and that this will involve various specific things such as complying with safety and hygienic measures including hand washing, it is not obvious that immunisation is a relevantly similar procedure. Indeed, one could argue that there is a clear difference between immunisation and hand washing, as vaccination is a procedure that interferes with one's bodily integrity in a way that hand washing does not. The notion of bodily integrity expresses the idea that each has a right to his own body, and a primary role in decisions about what may happen to it. This implies that others are prohibited from harming a person's body without his explicit consent. It also implies that we should respect the privacy of a person's body; we simply cannot commandeer or use another person's body. Immunisation is thus a more invasive action than hand washing. Health care workers can consider it 'too much' when they are required to be immunised against the flu in order to protect others.

One can also object that the boundaries between one's private and professional spheres of life will fade away when immunisation is held to be part of one's professional responsibilities. One cannot leave one's immunization behind at work, and one cannot neglect one's personal concerns towards influenza illness when deliberating about an immunisation request. For example, a health care worker who does not mind having the flu now and then, because it is not life threatening to healthy adults, suddenly has to decide whether she really wants to reduce the chance of becoming ill.

Even more, we may wonder whether a policy of mandatory immunisation would be disrespectful to health care professionals, because one would make 'instrumental use' of their bodies in order to protect frail residents.

Cost can 'surpass' the individual as well. Mandatory immunisation can change the profession in such ways that individuals within that practice can conclude that these changing responsibilities and demands change their profession in a negative way. They may experience a gap between the initial practice they once entered and the actual current responsibilities imposed upon them. To illustrate this argument we can point out that increasing knowledge about health determinants enables us to protect and stimulate our health in multiple new ways. As a result, in much health care practice we see a shift in focus from caring towards preventive measures and activities. Besides the fact that new activities will involve new and different responsibilities for health care workers, to which they may not feel optimally equipped, for many preventive aims it is true that they can be stimulated in multiple and various different ways. Health care professionals might fear that their responsibilities to prevent infections could become limitless if they were expected to live up to the general preventive aim in the best way they can. Moreover, prevention does not relate directly to an actual disease but the chance that one will become ill. If we realise that the health and well-being of residents can be stimulated in endless ways, it can seem a rather arbitrary choice to insist upon the immunisation of nursing home staff when most residents do not receive enough nutrition or liquids, or are immobilised and hardly ever get outside anymore. Why should a health care worker be motivated to get vaccinated if these other issues are not given any attention?

8.4. Demandingness and Reasonable Morality

Both the arguments that speak in favour of special responsibilities of health care workers as well as the arguments that reject mandatory immunisation policies aim to discuss the question—what will be a reasonable request of health care professionals? On the one hand, I argued, we can expect them to make an extra effort to stimulate the health and well-being of residents and to ward off outbreaks of influenza, while on the other hand, some limits may have to be respected if we want to avoid the idea that an immunisation request may become too burdensome.

I think that some of the considerations that I presented as possible burdens to agents could even be accepted as a 'cost to the agent', that is, as a morally relevant factor that can outweigh or block other considerations that speak in favour of immunisation. Such 'costs' mainly depend on two conditions being fulfilled. First, whether within an ethical theoretical framework these factors will be recognized and accepted as relevant consideration. Second, it also depends on the status that can be given to such considerations within that same theoretical outlook. In this section, I will address the issue as to how a consideration regarding a potential burden to an agent can become accepted or rejected as a relevant moral consideration, and I will make use of two ethical theories to illustrate this point.

If my argument is convincing, it will also support the commonsense ideas about reasonableness that I presented in section two. Moreover, if one accepts that issues of reasonableness play a role in the influenza immunisation case, it also shows that our ideas of reasonable demands are not limited to extreme policies like the one-child policy in China or very stringent measures to prevent the spread of a deadly virus.[6] The consequence will be that many public health activities may be open to critique in the sense that such policies and preventive measures will need to be reasonable from an agent's point of view.

8.4.1. Act-Utilitarianism

From a welfarist consequentialist perspective, such an act-utilitarian view, the outcomes of actions are the primary relevant normative factor. Within

---

[6] Think of SARS or the risks of bird flu to human beings.

this perspective it is possible to accept that something can be burdensome to an agent, but what is conceived as burdensome is often limited to considerations of well-being. As a result, the commonsense arguments that I presented in section two will be accepted only as long as the 'burdens' relate to considerations of well-being. Thus, having to forego one's special commitments to a friend or the frustrating effects of endless responsibilities must affect one's well-being or otherwise these considerations are not accepted as relevant.

With respect to our case, we can see that this focus on well-being prevents us accepting specific considerations that could have been brought to the fore by opponents of mandatory immunisation. Disrespecting health care workers because one makes instrumental use of their bodies, or the fading away of boundaries between one's private and professional roles, as well as the fact that one can no longer feel comfortable with increasing and new responsibilities, will be accepted less easily as relevant considerations in relation to what is burdensome to the agent. As a matter of fact, a straightforward balancing of reasons will lead to the conclusion that there are only mild effects to agents, and that this certainly cannot outweigh the possible benefits to the residents.

Even if we would accept a broad notion of consequences within this view, and are willing to accept boundaries that do respect limits to, for example, the instrumental use of a person's body, it would still be hard to accept that these considerations could block or silence other considerations, so that they would prevail over the benefit to the residents of health care worker immunisation. Instead, a consequentialist will be more inclined to accept each of these considerations as only being one amongst many, and that the weighing of all considerations will lead to the best overall judgement. Thus, if expected benefit to residents are impressive, or when a great number of residents will benefit from the immunisation of the home personnel—that is if we accept an aggregative argument—the burdensome effects on agents will certainly be outweighed.[7]

We see that the perspective on what can be accepted as burdensome to agents is narrowly focused in this perspective, and that there is no inclination to accept 'cost to the agent' as a relevant moral consideration. On this view, such a 'cost' cannot be held to be a self-standing normative factor that can block or silence other considerations.

---

[7] Aggregation is a means to sum the burdens or benefits across individuals and claim that this sum carries moral weight. This is a strategy that is frequently embraced within consequentialism, but is open to dispute.

8.4.2. Contractualism

We can reach a different conclusion if we turn to another ethical theoretical perspective. Scanlon has recently defined the contours of a contractualist view in which the central moral question is held to be what people are obligated to do in relation to each other (Scanlon 1998). According to Scanlon, we should not focus on the outcome of our actions, but on what we can justify to all other participants in the moral community, because we want to stand in mutual respecting relationships with other people. We will accept those principles and rules that no one can reasonably reject (Scanlon 1998: 33). What will be reasonably acceptable to each participant in a deliberation process will depend on what from her point of view will be the consequences of a specific rule or principle, and when this seems unacceptable, this could lead to a reasonable objection to that principle.

We can expect that a contractualist framework will be more open to other types of considerations than a consequentialist framework that focuses only on considerations of well-being. Contractualists can recognize an agent's frustration, because this might imply that one is disrespectful to the other as a moral agent when endless demands are made on him. Or it will be disrespectful to an agent to expect him to breach moral rules that he embraces wholeheartedly.

With respect to the influenza immunisation case, this leads to the following picture. A contractualist framework will be more open to the objection that mandatory immunisation will lead to the instrumental use of a person's body, because it is disrespectful to other human beings to use them instrumentally. In a similar way, they could be more susceptible to considerations that involve the frustrating effects of cumulating responsibilities and the possible intrusion in one's bodily integrity. Moreover, such considerations could be highly relevant when we consider that contractualism does not only focus on the judgements we make in a single case, but generalizes each decision by asking whether a world in which it would be common practice to make instrumental use of others should be preferred.[8] If this can be reasonably rejected, this is sufficient to block the acceptance of such a principle.

What would a contractualist conclude with respect to the influenza immunisation case? Will it simply accept each objection and reject the idea

---

[8] Kumar (2001) stresses this several times in his presentation of the contractualist framework.

of mandatory immunisation? We could come to this conclusion, but only after we have given equal thought to each participant in the deliberation process. After all, if the basic interests of residents are at stake, they could, from their point of view, reasonably object to the rejection of a principle requiring mandatory immunisation. Depending on the relevant data and circumstances either the objections from health care workers or the claim of residents to get optimal protection from the flu will be a reasonable demand.

This brief outline of different ethical perspectives sketches only the contours, not the depths, of a difference in focus and how this focus will determine what will be recognized and accepted as a relevant consideration. I wanted to point out that this could lead to a completely different picture. Hence, when we discuss what will be a reasonable demand upon agents, we cannot escape the question about what ethical theoretical framework this is deliberated within.

We can also expect that one's ethical theoretical outlook will influence one's view on what will be a reasonable demand. An act-utilitarian will simply have a different view to a contractualist on this matter when we apply this to the influenza immunisation case. However, if we want to take seriously the claims that are made from a commonsense perspective, and conceive these commonsense ideas as widely shared beliefs in society, we should avoid becoming too alienated from the commonsense ideas about reasonableness, and be prepared to broaden the scope of what counts as being burdensome to agents. Otherwise we risk finding that agents will no longer be motivated and lose interest in complying with their moral responsibilities.

8.5. Relevance to Public Health Debates

Public health programmes are highly dependent on the compliance, and motivation, of individual agents. We apparently hold some ideas in common about what would be an unreasonable demand on agents, and some extreme measures, even to fight the disastrous effects of overpopulation, are intuitively rejected as too burdensome. However, the influenza immunisation case, a fairly simple and not often disputed issue, shows that in a less extreme case, questions about the reasonableness of a demand upon agents can also be discussed. If agents consider that the line of reasonableness is crossed and a specific request will be too burdensome on them, this will influence their willingness to comply. Moreover, if agents consider something as too burdensome, it is not their motivation that is lacking, but the fact that there are huge sacrifices involved that will explain why an agent is reluctant to comply; it is simply 'too much' from his perspective. Thus, public health programmes are urged to take the notion of reasonableness into consideration.

From a public health ethics perspective, we can insist that reasonableness should be taken into account and that two reasons support this idea. First, our commonsense ideas about reasonableness and burdens to agents involve a variety of considerations. These different considerations are recognized and acknowledged in different ethical theories. That is, when we analyse a case from different ethical perspectives, what will be recognized as burdensome will differ with the theoretical outlook that one takes. But all these considerations seem related to the commonsense arguments that I presented in section two. This urges us, therefore to broaden our scope and allow for different considerations that discuss the demandingness of moral obligations and responsibilities—and in our case of the moral considerations supporting public health programmes and activities.

Second, if burdens to agents are somehow accepted as a relevant moral consideration, we are also stimulated to (re)consider the status of these burdens in our moral deliberations. Should we accept a notion of 'cost to the agent' that can possibly block, silence or outweigh other considerations? And if so, we should seriously consider what the effects would be on public health programmes and activities. It will at least imply that the collective aims that we try to achieve do not go through without discussion, but that we seriously have to deliberate about the burdens and sacrifices that will fall upon agents. If burdens should be viewed as broadly as the commonsense view suggests, this could go far beyond the burdens of a—technical—intervention and effects on an agent's well-being and we should become more susceptible to other serious effects on agents.

9

Vertical Transmission of Infectious Diseases and Genetic Disorder: Are the Medical and Public Responses Consistent?

Jay A. Jacobson, Margaret P. Battin, Jeffrey R. Botkin, Leslie Francis, James O. Mason, and Charles B. Smith

Transmissible infectious diseases differ from most other diseases, not only by their etiology but by the risk they pose to others. Public policy, law, and ethics acknowledge this distinction by limiting the autonomy and diagnostic and treatment choices of individuals who potentially threaten others. For example, we may require patients with tuberculosis to wear a mask in the hospital. We may insist that they take their daily medicine under direct observation. If they refuse treatment, we may limit their movements to reduce exposure to others. Similarly, we have isolated patients with SARS and quarantined individuals who were exposed to this infection. We may require that children be immunized against several infectious diseases before they begin school. This contrasts with the freedom of action and medical choice accorded to persons with other kinds of disease even if their conditions pose a great threat to themselves. Thus, there seem to be two ethical paradigms operating here. The first, a utilitarian approach, limits individual liberty to maximize the greater good by ensuring the safety of many others. The second, a deontological view, places its greatest emphasis on the principle of autonomy, regardless of health consequences to the patient and society. The autonomy based paradigm generally requires voluntary treatment policies, whereas in situations where disease poses a significant risk to others, the utilitarian paradigm would favor coercive or compulsory treatment.

Transmission of infectious diseases can be from person to person. This can occur in two directions. The first is horizontal, which results from direct or indirect contact between persons. The second is vertical, which results from an infection passed from mother to fetus. Examples include syphilis and Human Immunodeficiency Virus (HIV) infection. Vertical transmission of disease is characteristic not only of infectious diseases, but also of genetic disorders. This shared characteristic invites us to examine how we think about and respond to different diseases and categories of disease that can be transmitted to our offspring. The policies that have emerged for infectious diseases and genetic disorders, both vertically transmitted, seem to be inconsistent. This divergence would be appropriate if there are morally relevant differences in these categories of disease, their treatments, or policies about how treatment is administered. In this chapter, we explore reasons that might explain or justify these apparently inconsistent policies.

Many examples of infectious diseases and genetic disorders might enable us to explore which ethical paradigm seems most appropriate and how medical care, public policy, and public health law have responded to the risk of vertical transmission—including syphilis, gonorrhea, hepatitis B, rubella, cystic fibrosis, Huntington's disease, phenylketonuria, sickle cell anemia, and Tay-Sach's disease, to name a few. In this chapter, we will focus on syphilis as an example of a vertically transmitted infectious disease and cystic fibrosis as a representative genetic disorder. We focus on syphilis and cystic fibrosis for three reasons. First, each is or has been relatively common. Second, we have known a good deal about their clinical manifestations and how to identify the disease and its cause for quite a long time (Quetel and Braddoch 1992; Shal 1996). Third, we can examine a substantial amount of public policy and written recommendations and practices associated with these examples (Morabia and Zhang 2004; Wilfond and Thomson 2000). We will compare these diseases with respect to their clinical manifestations, epidemiology, morbidity, and mortality. We will also explore our abilities to diagnose, treat, and prevent the diseases themselves and the tools we have to identify the causative agent or gene. We will review the medical and public health responses to each, with special attention to the strategies available for prevention and how and when they are used.

Because we think the responses to infectious and genetic vertical transmission may be inconsistent, we will consider their social and historical context and the responses to another vertically transmitted disease, HIV infection, to help us identify possible reasons or justifications for the inconsistency. We recognize that many experts in medical and public health ethics have proposed that genetic disorders should be treated in a special fashion partly because of their implications for genetically related individuals in addition to children (National Institutes of Health 2000). Others have pointed out that there are not sufficient distinctions between genetic and nongenetic tests to justify 'genetic exceptionalism' (Green and Botkin 2003). Our focus on vertical transmission, the key distinguishing feature of genetic disorders, allows us to examine whether vertical transmission merits special consideration or whether there is something else about genetic diseases (or infections) that warrants a special or exceptional approach.

Table 9.1. Definitions

Infectious Disease—A condition caused by biological agent.

Communicable Infectious Disease—A condition caused by a biological agent that can be transmitted from person to person.

Genetic Disorder—An abnormal health or physical condition attributed to the combined action of genes and the environment.

Inherited Genetic Disorder (Genetic Disease)—An abnormal health or physical condition that results from the passage of deleterious genes from parents to fetus.

Vertical Transmission—The transmission of infectious disease, pathogen, genetic disorder, or deleterious genes from one generation to another. This can occur *in-utero* for both types of diseases. For infectious diseases it may also occur intra-partum by exposure to blood and secretions or post-partum by exposure to breast milk.

Carrier—A person who shows no symptoms of the disease but who harbors the infectious agent of that disease and can transmit it and transmit it vertically or a person that carries one gene for a particular recessive trait and does not express the trait, but when mated with another carrier, can produce offspring who do.

9.1. Syphilis

The manifestations of syphilis have been recognized since the time of Hippocrates. The first recognized outbreak, however, occurred in Naples, in 1494, and involved a number of Spaniards from Christopher Columbus's crew who participated in the army of Charles the VIII of France (Tramont 2004). Shortly thereafter, people realized that the children of mothers with syphilis were adversely affected at birth. Congenital syphilis is a severe, disabling, and often life threatening condition for the infant. Nearly half of all children infected with syphilis during gestation die shortly before or after birth. Infants who survive develop early and late stage symptoms of syphilis if not treated. Early stage symptoms include irritability, failure to thrive, and non-specific fever. Some infants develop a rash and lesions on the mouth, anus, and genitalia. Some of these lesions may resemble the wart-like lesions of adult syphilis. A small percentage of infants have a watery nasal discharge and a saddle nose deformity resulting from infection in the cartilage of the nose. Bone lesions are common, especially in the upper arm. Later signs appear as tooth abnormalities, bone changes, neurological involvement, blindness, and deafness (US National Library and National Institute of Health 2004).

In the early 20th century in the United States, approximately one million women of childbearing age had syphilis. Congenital syphilis was the leading cause of spontaneous abortions and stillbirths. About twenty-five thousand fetuses per year died before birth and sixty thousand per year were born with syphilis. Between forty and one hundred percent of the fetuses carried by women with syphilis were infected. Since 1906, clinicians have been able to identify individuals infected with syphilis by using microscopy, which reveals the infectious agent, *Treponema pallidum*, in primary and cutaneous lesions and by a serologic test which identifies antibodies to the pathogen during latent infection and secondary or tertiary stages (Stoto et al. 1999: 26). Individuals may be carriers of this pathogen for years if they are untreated. Since the 1940s, penicillin has been used to effectively treat syphilis in all of its stages. Infants born to infected mothers who received adequate penicillin treatment during pregnancy are at minimal risk (Tramont 2005: 2781).

Numerous strategies are effective in preventing the vertical transmission of syphilis and reducing the consequences to infected fetuses if transmission has occurred. These strategies include premarital testing of men and women and treatment of either or both partners who have a positive test. Prenatal testing of pregnant women is another option. Treatment of an infected woman during pregnancy prevents and/or treats infection in the fetus. Postnatal or newborn screening of infants does not prevent syphilis, but early treatment of infected infants can reduce morbidity (Walker and Walker 2002).

9.2. Cystic Fibrosis

The syndrome of cystic fibrosis has been recognized since the middle ages, when infants with salty skin where considered 'bewitched' because they routinely died an early death. The syndrome was named 'cystic fibrosis with bronchiectasis' by Fanconi in 1936. In 1949, Lowe established it as a recessive genetic disorder and, by 1953, a more precise test for sweat chloride, the quantitative version of 'salty skin', became available for diagnosis. This enabled better diagnosis and characterization of the clinical syndrome. Cystic fibrosis manifests its symptoms in early infancy and childhood. It is characterized by recurrent bouts of pneumonia, failure to thrive, and pancreatic insufficiency. Most males with cystic fibrosis are infertile. Only about 40% of children with cystic fibrosis live beyond age eighteen. The average life span for those who live to adulthood is thirty to thirty-three years. Death is usually from pulmonary complications (US Department of Energy 2002).

Cystic fibrosis is the most common fatal hereditary disorder affecting Caucasians in the United States. It is most common among Caucasians of Northern or Central European descent. Clinical risk factors include a family history of cystic fibrosis or unexplained infant death. Cystic fibrosis is an autosomal recessive disorder. Thus a child must receive an abnormal gene from both parents to be affected. The carrier rate for Americans for the single abnormal gene is approximately one in twenty. There are approximately twelve million carriers in the United States. The likelihood that two Caucasian carriers will marry and/or mate is approximately one in four hundred. Because the disease is transmitted as an autosomal recessive, 50% of their offspring will be carriers, 25% will inherit neither abnormal gene, and 25% will inherit both abnormal genes and probably develop the disease. This results in an annual incidence of approximately one in sixteen hundred births to Caucasians and one in four thousand total births in the United States (US Department of Energy 2002).

There is no curative treatment for cystic fibrosis. However early recognition and treatment can lengthen survival and improve quality of life. Treatment includes antibiotic, enzymes, vitamins, and bronchodilators. New treatments included replacement of the DNAse enzyme with Dornase (Pulmozyme). Genetic research hopes to correct the disease by artificially inserting a 'normal' gene into the affected person. An intranasal form of this gene therapy is currently undergoing clinical trials. Research on methods that could treat the disorder before birth seems promising (Littlewood 2002).

Strategies for preventing cystic fibrosis consist of identifying carriers and having those carriers exercise available reproductive choices. Carriers can be identified by a blood test for the CFTR gene. This test can be done as a premarital screen. At that point couples can consider options to prevent the birth of a child with CF. If they would consider abortion of an affected fetus, they can choose to have prenatal testing of the fetus with chorionic villus sampling (CVS). They could choose *in vitro* fertilization and selective implantation of an unaffected embryo. They could use artificial insemination with sperm from a non-carrier. They could choose to adopt.

9.3. Strategies for Testing for these Two Vertically Transmitted Diseases

Prenatal syphilis testing was available by 1906, but was not mandated by law due to 'onerous treatment options and the stigma of being shown to have the disease'. Indeed, even being tested for syphilis was stigmatizing, and many physicians were reluctant to embarrass women in their care by suggesting it. In 1936, Thomas Parran, the US Surgeon General, established a program that included mandatory premarital and prenatal blood tests. By the end of 1945, thirty-six states had passed prenatal syphilis screening laws. Under these laws, birth certificates had to record whether the test had been done prenatally and to explain why those who were not tested were not. Women and physicians could refuse on religious or other grounds. Although these laws were passed before the introduction of antibiotic treatment, they resulted in a rapid decline of congenital transmission through case finding, contact tracing, and the difficult and less effective therapies available at the time. Perhaps the most important aspect of these screening programs was that by making testing routine, they overcame the resistance of physicians to risk offending patients by suggesting a test for syphilis (Stoto et al. 1999).

These control measures were so effective that, as of 2004, fewer than five states continue to require premarital testing because the frequency of positive results is so low. However, forty-six of fifty states still require prenatal testing of pregnant women. 76% of states that mandate testing require one early test and 26% require a second later test for all or high-risk women (Hollier et al. 2003). In situations where the test is mandated, written informed consent is not usually solicited. Thirty-three states allow religious exemption from testing and thirteen permit refusal for any reason. Insurance generally covers the cost of testing if a bill is generated, but many clinics that do this test do not charge for it. By supporting the infrastructure to deliver prenatal screening, state laws do indirectly influence practice. Many state antepartum screening laws, for example, have misdemeanor penalties for violations, and some states offer laboratory testing at reduced or no cost (General Accounting Office 2003).

Physician practice is influenced not only by state law but also by professional society recommendations. Current guidelines from the American College of Obstetrics and Gynecology and the American Academy of Pediatrics recommend that all women be screened for syphilis at the first prenatal visit; women considered to be at high risk for the disease should be screened again at thirty two to thirty six weeks gestation (American Academy of Pediatrics 2002).

As a result of these policies—and practices that are in relatively good compliance with them—new syphilis cases in the United States in 2002 fell to 32, 871. New primary and secondary syphilis cases had an incidence of 2.4 per 100,000 population. Prevalence of carriers among woman was one per hundred thousand. The total number of cases of congenital syphilis was 451, for a rate of 11.2 cases per hundred thousand live births. The total number of cases of congenital syphilis decreased from the 492 reported in 2001 (CDC 2002b, 2003).

In addition to recommendations to practitioners, medical professional societies also offer guidance to women to prevent vertical transmission of syphilis. They say to women:

If you suspect that you may be infected with syphilis and are pregnant or anticipate becoming pregnant, call your health care provider immediately. Safer sexual practices can help prevent infection. If you suspect you have syphilis, seek medical attention immediately to avoid complications like infecting a fetus during pregnancy or birth. Prenatal care for expectant mothers is critical. During prenatal care evaluations, a routine serologic test for syphilis is done. This identifies infected mothers and allows them to be treated to minimize the risk to the infant and to themselves.

(US National Library of Medicine and National Institute of Health 2004)

With respect to cystic fibrosis, we know that screening of family members of a cystic fibrosis patient may detect a cystic fibrosis gene in between 60% and 90% of carriers, depending upon the test used. Similarly, if the test were used in Caucasians who do not have a family member with cystic fibrosis, it could be expected to identify the majority of carriers, with the precision depending upon the test used (National Institutes of Health 1997).

Policies regarding cystic fibrosis stand in significant contrast to these policies regarding syphilis. No states require premarital or prenatal screening for cystic fibrosis. The American College of Obstetricians and Gynecologists (ACOG) now recommends that the carrier-screening test be available to all couples that are planning pregnancy or are pregnant (American College of Obstetricians and Gynecologists 2001). Many healthcare providers hand out printed material for the couples to read. Those who may be interested in testing can then discuss it further with their providers.

The National Institutes of Health, in a consensus development conference statement in 1997, made several recommendations. They stated that individuals with a family history of CF and partners of those with CF should be offered genetic testing. CF genetic testing should be offered to the prenatal population and couples currently planning a pregnancy, particularly those in high-risk populations. CF testing for the general population is not advocated. Genetic testing for CF should begin with education concerning CF. It should be clear that the patient has received the material and has had an opportunity for questions to be answered before testing is undertaken. All persons undergoing genetic testing should give written informed consent for the test, receive culturally sensitive educational materials, and demonstrate an understanding of the test and the test results (National Institutes of Health 1997).

Genetic testing and interpretation of test results are complex. A couple in which both partners are carriers should consider consulting a genetic counselor, who can discuss the risks to their future children. A genetic counselor can discuss the option of prenatal testing (using amniocentesis or CVS) to diagnosis or rule out CF in the fetus. Whether or not a couple chooses to take the carrier-screening test is a personal decision. A couple must decide whether it is right for them after learning more about CF and discussing the test with their healthcare provider. Newborn testing for CF does not directly prevent vertical transmission. However, rapid diagnosis of the genetic condition in the neonate may lead to earlier appropriate treatment, which may be life extending and enhancing. It could also lead indirectly to parental choices, which might prevent or address vertical transmission in subsequent pregnancies.

According to the NIH, the direct costs for treating cystic fibrosis are forty thousand dollars per year per patient. The ancillary costs are nine thousand dollars per year. Using a 3% discount rate, this implies a net present value of approximately eight hundred thousand dollars for direct and ancillary costs associated with a CF birth. Studies have shown that the hypothetical costs per identified CF fetus averted ranged from two hundred fifty thousand dollars to one million two hundred fifty thousand dollars for Caucasian population of Northern European ancestry (National Institutes of Health 1997). The moral relevance of these costs is controversial. They could provide reasons for medical insurers including the state to promote cost saving practices. If potential parents were financially responsible, the costs could have a substantial effect on their decisions as well.

While states have not yet reported the results of voluntary or recommended testing with respect to CF births, there is a recent report from a large healthcare organization in California. 'The nation's largest prenatal [during early pregnancy] cystic fibrosis screening program identified two thousand three carriers of CF gene mutations in its first four years and resulted in the births of half the expected number of babies with the disease' (Bates 2003).

9.4. Syphilis and Cystic Fibrosis Compared

These two vertically transmitted disorders are similar with respect to severity of disease, potential incidence, detectability of cases, and carriers, and the absence of curative treatment after vertical transmission occurs, but there are substantial differences in strategies for prevention. An inexpensive, safe drug, penicillin, can be used to prevent vertical transmission of syphilis. Only reproductive choices are available to prevent vertical transmission of cystic fibrosis. The types of regulation, policy and practice differ in dramatic ways as well. Public policy enables and strongly promotes prevention of vertical transmission for syphilis, although when transmitted it can be a less serious disease. However, policies emphasize parental choice for prevention of cystic fibrosis, although cystic fibrosis almost always results in a shortened lifespan for affected offspring. In the case of cystic fibrosis,

> every attempt should be made to protect the individual rights, genetic and medical privacy rights, and to prevent discrimination and stigmatization. It is essential that the offering of CF carrier testing be phased in over a period of time to insure that adequate education and appropriate genetic testing and counseling services are available to all persons being tested.

> (National Institutes of Health 1997)

Past and present screening policies for syphilis can be characterized as preconception, prenatal, paternalistic, state mandated, universal, with presumed consent for tests and treatment, widely practiced, and effective. Screening policies for cystic fibrosis can be characterized as prenatal, postnatal, selective, and voluntary. Cystic fibrosis screening stresses autonomous, informed, voluntary choices and neutral counseling; syphilis testing is, in effect, mandatory.

9.5. What would Explain these Differences?

The history, cultures and practices of those who do genetic medicine and counseling are different from those who specialize in public health. However, there may be other, perhaps more morally relevant, reasons for the differences in policies. Prenatal testing for syphilis began in an era of paternalism, and screening for cystic fibrosis in an era of patient rights and autonomy. There is cheap, easy, effective treatment and prevention for syphilis, which invites universal testing. The nature of the prevention strategies for cystic fibrosis, both the expense of some reproductive strategies and the controversial nature of abortion may deter government mandates and the wide practice of voluntary testing. Because the chance of vertical transmission in the case of syphilis ranges from 40% to 100% (Bale 2002) but in the case of cystic fibrosis is only 25% this conceivably could diminish public pressure and personal preference for prevention. Especially if the only preventive measures are avoidance of conception, selective conception via assisted reproductive technology, or abortion, and these strategies may be particularly expensive or potentially violate strongly held personal or religious positions.

It may be helpful to review six principles of public health screening and consider how they apply to the two disorders we have discussed. The principles are:

1. Goals are specified and achievable;
2. Natural history is known and intervention effective;
3. Screening tests are without high false positives or negatives;
4. Adequate diagnosis and treatment of true positives is possible;
5. Tests and interventions are acceptable to affected population; and
6. Cost of case finding, diagnosis, and intervention are reasonable in relation to benefits and other programs.

(Wilson and Jungner 1968; Stoto et al. 1999: 22–3)

With respect to the first principle, the goal would seem to be prevention of congenital syphilis in infants. A seemingly similar goal is possible in the case of cystic fibrosis, but achievable only through expensive and, to some, ethically troubling reproductive choices. However, in the case of syphilis, the goal may be more specifically stated as the prevention of disease, or a known harm, in an existing fetus, which continues to develop until delivery. For cystic fibrosis, however, at present the achievable goal should be more precisely stated as the prevention not of harm to the fetus, but as prevention of conception or the development of affected fetuses, or more starkly, the prevention of birth of affected infants: It is simply not yet possible to have *this* child without cystic fibrosis.[1] These two goals then are very different. One reason to screen is to prevent harm to a fetus. A second reason to screen is to prevent the birth. This different goal for CF is unlikely to achieve the same level of public and government support. With respect to principles two and three, the two disorders are quite similar. However, with respect to principle four, there is adequate diagnosis of both diseases and carrier states but while there is simple, cheap and effective treatment for syphilis, there is less effective

[1] For a discussion of what has come to be called the 'non-identity' problem, see McMahan (2002: § 8.2). From an impersonal point of view, it may be better for a non-affected child to be born than for an affected child to be born. See, e.g., Purdy (1999). From the point of view of an affected child, however, abortion cannot be better; the only alternative to being born with CF is not to be born at all.

drug treatment for cystic fibrosis. Regarding principle five, the simple, cheap tests and interventions for syphilis do appear to be quite acceptable to the general and the affected population. It is still difficult to say on a national level how acceptable the tests and interventions are to Caucasians for cystic fibrosis. However, although they were not asked specifically about syphilis or cystic fibrosis, in an Office of Technology Assessment survey over a decade ago, 83% of Americans said they would take a genetic test before having children, if it would tell them whether their children would likely inherit a fatal genetic disease (National Institutes of Health 1997).

With respect to principle six, the cost of case and carrier finding and intervention to prevent vertical transmission has been cost effective for syphilis, but is, of course, prevalence dependent. Case and carrier finding for cystic fibrosis could be cost effective in the Caucasian population in the United States with its present carrier prevalence, but only if a significant proportion of informed parents choose strategies that avoid the birth of an affected infant.

Thus, we see that with respect to six principles that could justify a relatively aggressive public health strategy, our knowledge and intervention strategies for syphilis and cystic fibrosis are quite similar, but are certainly not identical. The critical differences lie in the specifically achievable goals and the means used to achieve them. This could explain and perhaps justify the differences in public policies that address prevention of these two disorders. From a utilitarian perspective, while the benefits of two strategies that both prevent the birth of affected infants may be similar, the burdens of the preventive strategies for cystic fibrosis, both perceived and actual, are quite different.

The second consideration, not apparent from a reference to principles, is the time and social environment in which each policy was introduced. The period after World War II was a time when it was understandably easy to portray syphilis as the enemy, to laud penicillin as a magic bullet, and to rally public support for a sustained campaign to attack syphilis and to protect its potential victims, especially children. Medical decision-making at that time would now be described as paternalistic, where physicians generally decided what was best for their patients. It is perhaps no surprise that patients, and even couples about to marry, accepted a near universal mandatory screening, treatment, and prenatal prevention approach. Currently, there are widely available tools for carrier and fetal case detection for cystic fibrosis and the legal and biological ways to initiate or terminate pregnancy, these emerged as medical paternalism was being challenged and displaced by civil

Table 9.2. Contrasts between Syphilis and Cystic Fibrosis

Syphilis	Cystic Fibrosis
Prenatal testing began in an era of paternalism.	Prenatal testing began in an era of autonomy.
There is inexpensive, effective treatment.	There is no preventative treatment for a conceived fetus.
The treatment is relatively easy.	Reproductive treatment strategies are expensive and ethically controversial, including only abortion, avoidance of conception, and selective conception via assisted reproductive technology.
The chance of vertical transmission is high, although variable, between 40 and 100 %.	The chance of vertical transmission is 25%.
The goal of screening is to prevent harm to the fetus.	The goal of screening is to prevent the birth of an affected developing fetus.
Case and carrier finding is cost effective.	Case and carrier finding could be cost effective only if a significant proportion of informed parents chose strategies that avoided the birth of an affected fetus.

rights, consumer rights, women's rights, gay rights, and patient's rights, as epitomized by the doctrine of informed consent and the current regard for patient autonomy.

Thus, these changes in the social environment, particularly emphasis on individual rights and choice, may be more important in explaining different strategies than that one type of vertical transmission is infectious and the other is genetic. The advent of HIV/AIDS in the early 1980s allows us to examine this thesis. We can do so because of the feared and stigmatized nature of this morbid and presumed fatal disease, the rapid evolution of diagnostic and screening tests, the recognition and quantification of vertical transmission, the lack of curative treatment, but especially because of the availability of interventions that reduce the risk of and even prevent vertical transmission.

In many ways, public health policy for prevention of this vertically transmitted infectious disease looks less like the policy we have for syphilis and more like our policy for cystic fibrosis. Despite an incidence of HIV infected newborns, (0.1–2 per 100), much greater than that for syphilis, (10–100 per 100,000) there is no required premarital or prenatal screening for HIV

(Saah 1996; CDC 2002c). When prenatal screening is offered, it is required to be absolutely voluntary and absolutely informed. There are even specially trained counselors, in some ways analogous to genetic counselors, who are often employed to perform this function. Similarly, as with cystic fibrosis, an array of reproductive choices is available to an HIV infected woman before and after a pregnancy begins. None of these choices have been mandated and the thrust of policy is that there be neither mandate nor coercion. However, as with syphilis, drugs can prevent maternal infant transmission of HIV before and/or during pregnancy. Mandatory testing and antiviral treatment of pregnant women would be consistent with policies for managing vertically transmitted syphilis, an infectious disease scourge of an earlier era. Nevertheless, in the current era, no policy mandates such treatment.

9.6. Inconsistencies in Policy Approaches to Vertically Transmitted Diseases

Thus, it appears not only that there are inconsistencies in our policy approach to vertically transmitted disease that seem to relate to the general classification of the disorder and to the nature of the preventative intervention, but there are also apparent inconsistencies in the way we address two vertically transmitted infectious diseases, syphilis and HIV. This may be more related to historical context and prevailing public expectations and religious and social mores than to material differences in the epidemiology, treatment, or prevention of the diseases.

If research produces, as it is likely to do, a safe, effective *in utero* treatment for a fetus that is homozygous for the CF gene, we will have another meaningful way to examine whether we use similar policies for similar disorders.

Even now it may not be too soon to consider whether we should approach the prevention of vertically transmitted HIV the way we approached syphilis or perhaps change, and update, our rather paternalistic approach to syphilis to conform with contemporary respect for individual patients' and particularly women's rights. If we do the latter, it should be with due regard for the remarkable success the present pregnancy-related and other aggressive preventive strategies have had in the virtual elimination of vertically transmitted syphilis.

However, in the case of HIV a change in medical interventions may also help to rationalize or resolve the current differences in public health policies. We must acknowledge that there is nothing akin to penicillin with respect to safety, inexpensiveness, and efficacy yet available for HIV infection. However, a curative drug or effective vaccine is at least conceivable. If either materializes we believe we can expect to see more aggressive public health policies *a la* syphilis and much better voluntary compliance with widely espoused, but not mandated recommendations to test and to treat. Until then, in an age of patient autonomy, we may expect to see social or ethical 'grandfathering' of earlier more paternalistic strategies.

10

Herd Protection as a Public Good: Vaccination and our Obligations to Others

Angus Dawson[1]

Many contagious diseases can result in serious harm and even death for the affected individuals. However, several of these diseases can be prevented through vaccination. In developed countries routine childhood vaccination policies have been successful in reducing the incidence of such diseases.[2] The World Health Organization and other bodies are extending such benefits to the developing world (WHO 2002c). However, many individuals, especially children, die each year from vaccine-preventable illness. I would argue that there are many ethical issues that arise in relation to this topic. However, the focus of this chapter is upon contagious diseases where an option exists

[1] Thanks to members of the following audiences for discussion of earlier versions of the arguments in this chapter: the Public Health and Ethical Theory seminar co-sponsored by the Netherlands School for Research in Practical Philosophy and the Netherlands Organization for Scientific Research, held at Bilthoven in the Netherlands (May 2002); vaccination ethics seminar at Gothenburg University, Sweden (May 2003); the MA in Applied Ethics seminar at Utrecht University in the Netherlands (March 2004); and to the seminar at Manchester University Philosophy Department (May 2004). I would particularly like to thank Marcel Verweij, Frans Brom, Yash Paul, Harry Lesser, Sorin Baiasu, and Daniel Hill for helpful comments.

[2] See, for example, the tables and discussion in Ulmer and Liu (2002) and the records of laboratory reports in relation to many contagious diseases in the UK presented in Salisbury and Begg (1996: passim).

to be vaccinated in advance with the aim of preventing infection from such a disease. I will defend the idea that the existence of herd protection through vaccination for at least some contagious diseases brings about an important public good. The creation and maintenance of this particular public good will be so significant (at least in relation to some diseases) that it can be used to justify a moral obligation to undergo participation in some vaccination programmes. However, I argue that the obligation to contribute in this way is much weaker once herd protection is attained in a population. Indeed, individuals might have reasonable grounds for opting out of such vaccination programmes once herd protection exists. I suggest that it looks difficult to argue (at least on standard liberal lines) that you have an obligation to be vaccinated even when you derive benefit from belonging to a population where such herd protection exists. More specifically I argue that neither harm to others considerations nor free-rider arguments can be used to justify such an obligation. These conclusions can be supported by both pragmatic and consequentialist reasons.

It should be noted at this early stage that my discussions in this chapter are limited to arguments about the requirements imposed upon us by moral obligations. I do not discuss the issue of what obligations might be imposed through law. This means that where a moral obligation exists, and an individual chooses to ignore it, no external sanction will follow (except perhaps disapproval or adverse comment from others). This can be contrasted with the consequences of ignoring a legal obligation, which may result in a criminal or civil penalty. For example, if a particular vaccination is legally compulsory, then failure to be vaccinated may result in a fine or detention. If vaccination is morally obligated, for, say, harm-to-others reasons, a failure to vaccinate is largely a matter for that individual's conscience.[3]

10.1. The Nature of Contagious Diseases and Vaccinations

Vaccination for many contagious diseases has two potentially positive outcomes. The first is that it provides some protection to the individual *qua*

---

[3] Of course, there will be some overlap between the arguments about moral and legal obligations to undergo vaccination. I hope to discuss the nature of such legal obligations elsewhere.

individual by raising the level of their personal immunity to a particular disease. The second is that it contributes to protection at the level of the group or population by increasing the general level of immunity within the relevant population, ensuring that an outbreak of that particular disease is less likely. Such a characteristic is generally called herd immunity. I will, however, refer to it as herd protection following the distinction proposed by Paul (2004). He suggests that there is an important difference to be drawn between herd immunity and herd protection. He argues that we should think of herd immunity as being brought about through the rise in immunity for a disease within a non-vaccinated population caused through the secondary spread of the agent used in the vaccination programme in the environment (by way of such things as faecal matter from those who have been vaccinated). In this situation non-vaccinated members of a population might still have some immunity to the disease in question.[4] Herd protection by contrast exists more as a parallel to quarantine, where the non-vaccinated are protected from exposure to the disease just because of the existence of high rates of vaccination for that disease in the population as a whole. The existence of herd protection in a community does not guarantee that individual members of that community will not come into contact with the relevant infectious agent. Herd protection protects the community because (where it exists) it is less likely that any infected individual will be able to pass on that disease within the relevant community. This is because where herd protection exists the vast majority of other individuals who come into contact with the infected individual, during the infectious period of the disease, already have immunity. As a result the disease is less likely to be maintained in that population and so epidemics are less likely to occur. This is also why different diseases require different percentages of the population to be vaccinated for herd protection to exist. Generally speaking, the more infectious the disease, and the longer the incubation period, the higher the percentage of the population needed to be vaccinated for herd protection to exist. Herd immunity in Paul's sense might raise some

---

[4] Perhaps the best example of this might be immunity created through the secondary spread of polio immunity through the use of Oral Poliovirus Vaccine (OPV). See Paul (2004) and Paul and Dawson (2005) for discussion of this case.

interesting ethical issues of its own,[5] but it is herd protection that I am interested in here.[6]

Vaccination for a contagious disease can, therefore, be seen as an act that not only has potential benefits for the individual themselves but as also making a contribution towards a collective benefit as everyone profits where herd protection exists in the population, including those that are not vaccinated (for whatever reason) and those who do not show sufficient immune response despite vaccination. One way to think of these two positive outcomes is as being both a private (or individual) and a public (or collective) good. A private good is a good that benefits only the individual concerned and a public good benefits all of the members of a group or population. It is because of such a shared population benefit from the existence of herd protection that we might think of the existence of such a state as being a public good. We can think of public goods in general, following Klosko, as being characterised by two main properties: nonexcludability and dependence upon cooperation by a large number of people (Klosko 1987). 'Nonexcludable goods' are those where no one can be excluded from the benefits of the existence of the relevant good, even when they have not contributed towards bringing it about.[7] This is the case where herd protection exists: the non-vaccinated benefit from the high immunity in the population. In addition, herd protection can only be generated through collaborative endeavour as it cannot be created, obtained or controlled by any individual acting alone. In addition to these two aspects of public goods suggested by Klosko I would add another proposed by

[5] For example, should we take account of such secondary consequences in the development of our vaccination policies? If we should, is this an objection to certain types of vaccines? For example, if someone has a principled objection to receiving vaccinations, say, for religious reasons does such secondary 'vaccination' present a problem?

[6] Another issue that I will not address here is what might count as relevant in determining what constitutes the relevant 'herd'. We might seek to protect a local or national population rather than looking at this from a global perspective. This is certainly a common strategy for nation states.

[7] An excludable good would be one created jointly where the benefits are only enjoyed by the participants themselves. Examples of excludable goods might include a library created by subscription open to private members or a private health insurance scheme. In such cases, contributing members control who benefits from their actions. By contrast, all of the relevant population benefit from the existence and maintenance of a public good whatever their views about whether or not they will personally benefit or whether or not it should be maintained.

Rawls (1971). He suggests that public goods must also be indivisible: that is, they cannot be broken down or divided up into individual or private goods to be distributed amongst the members of a group or population. As we have seen, this is true of herd protection in the sense that the equal collective benefit can only come about as a result of collective action. Herd protection where it exists can therefore be seen to be a public good as it is indivisible, nonexcludable and dependent upon the cooperative actions of a group.[8]

The empirical facts relating to each disease and potential vaccine make a difference to many of the ethical arguments about vaccinations and this can be illustrated by considering a few examples. Diphtheria is an infection of the upper respiratory tract or the skin. It is usually fatal if left untreated. The disease is now so rare in the developed world, as a result of routine childhood vaccination since the 1940s, (Salisbury and Begg 1996: 68) that it has largely disappeared from public consciousness in many parts of the world although there have been recent severe outbreaks in the former Soviet Union (Garrett 2001). Polio provides another example of a disease that is extremely rare worldwide thanks to a successful vaccination campaign. The disease can cause permanent paralysis and death. Most vaccination programmes for contagious diseases such as those for diphtheria and polio potentially produce both private and public goods. However, this is not always the case. For example, some vaccination programmes do not produce a private good for all participating parties. A good example of a vaccination programme with a clear emphasis upon the production of a public good rather than private goods is routine childhood vaccination for rubella. This is a minor illness for most affected parties except for the effects upon a foetus during pregnancy. Permanent sensory and cognitive deprivation can be caused to the resultant child in such circumstances. It might be argued that for this particular disease vaccinating all children can only be justified if we create the public good of herd protection, thereby protecting the unborn. The vaccinated individuals will derive no (or only marginal) private good from the vaccination. Such a policy has of course benefits for all of those in the relevant society by reducing the number of children, brothers and sisters, and so on, damaged by such a disease (as well as benefiting us all through

---

[8] A more substantive list of features of public goods is given by many authors such as Cullity (1995). However, the characterisation given here is sufficient for the needs of the argument in this chapter.

cutting the costs of care for those affected). My point is that this is a policy primarily aimed at producing a population benefit rather than one focused on the individual. By contrast some other routine vaccinations are for diseases that while potentially harmful, and even deadly, are not contagious at all. The best example of such a disease is tetanus. Vaccination for tetanus can be seen to produce only a private good. This is because herd protection cannot be created for this disease as it cannot be transmitted between persons and the bacteria that cause the disease are prevalent in the environment.

The individual may therefore derive both a private good and a share in a public good through participation in at least some vaccination programmes. Those that are not vaccinated also derive benefit from the public good, even though they have not contributed to it through their own vaccination. In at least some of these cases this is because the individual cannot be vaccinated by virtue of the fact that there is some medical reason for non-vaccination, they are allergic to one or more component of the vaccine, or they are too young. In other cases it might be that individuals missed some or all of the available vaccinations because they were not registered with the relevant medical services or were elsewhere (perhaps even in a different country) at the scheduled times for vaccination. Such situations might be thought of as non-intentional non-vaccination. However, it is also possible that non-vaccination might be intentional as a result of a competent choice of the individual (or the choice of their parents where we are talking about children).[9] In this chapter I will focus on the situation where a competent adult individual has deliberately opted out of a vaccination programme.[10] I want to consider what moral obligations such an individual has to others in relation to vaccinations. I will argue that we should distinguish our obligations depending upon whether or not herd protection exists. The general issue to be explored is the degree to which it makes sense to suggest we have a moral obligation to undergo vaccination where an individual wishes to opt

[9] Whilst some parents explicitly refuse vaccinations for their children on religious, ideological, or 'risk'-related grounds, at least some non-vaccination of children is due to social and economic factors (Dare 1998).

[10] The issues will differ where we are thinking about third parties (e.g. parents) opting out of vaccination programme on behalf of others. We tend to think that parents will attempt to secure what is best for the child although this is not always the case. For the sake of a clearer focus to the discussion in this chapter the issues arising from such cases will be largely ignored here. However see Dawson (2005) for some discussion of 'best interests' in relation to childhood vaccinations.

out of a vaccination programme. I will consider two possible ways of arguing that such obligations can perhaps be legitimately imposed in such cases. The first argument appeals to the fundamental obligation to not cause harm to others and the second is based upon the idea of justice and suggests that we consider an opting-out from such vaccinations as a form of free-riding.

10.2. Harm to Others

Many writers have considered the bringing about of harm to others as an important reason not to perform certain acts. The first thing we need to consider is how we can fill out this supposed obligation in a little more detail. There are a number of different options here. The most obvious is to appeal to the popular moral principle of non-maleficence (Beauchamp and Childress 2001). The usual interpretation given to this principle is a narrow one: that is we are morally required to do no harm. In essence, this requires us to perform no action that creates harm. What exactly the concept 'harm' involves is surprisingly difficult to pin down (Feinberg 1973). I won't enter the debate about the exact nature of harm here, except to say that certain paradigm cases of harm are clear: causing pain, bringing about disability or death etc.

Most discussion of non-maleficence focuses on harm that has been created intentionally. However, harm can result from a failure to perform an action, as well as from an action. If I can act to prevent or remove the occurrence of harm, do I have a moral obligation to do so? If such an obligation exists, is it one of non-maleficence? Let's take the second question first. Once again the issue is open to debate. Those who wish to draw a sharp(ish) distinction between non-maleficence and beneficence argue that we can distinguish the two, and the obligation to prevent or remove harm is one of beneficence and not non-maleficence.[11] advocates of such a view may then go on to suggest that obligations of non-maleficence may be different in kind or take priority over those of beneficence.[12] Others suggest that obligations not to

[11] For example, Beauchamp and Childress argue for such a distinction (2001: 113–16).

[12] Once again, there may be different views on this issue. It might be the case that these principles are seen as being prima facie in nature, in which case non-maleficence will only

cause harm, to prevent harm, and to remove harm are all aspects of a single principle (Frankena 1973).[13] Again, I won't enter in this debate here, as my argument does not turn on this issue. However, this section does focus on the obligations relating to causing, failing to prevent or to remove harm, and of failing to reduce the risk of harm. I will refer to this class of issues as falling under an obligation not to bring about harm to others. I trust that we can remain neutral as to whether such obligations derive from principles of non-maleficence or beneficence and can just refer to this set of related obligations as the 'harm to others principle' (HOP). This principle will then be used to suggest the existence of a moral obligation to undergo vaccination in at least some situations.[14]

It should be noted that HOP is of course related to the harm to others principle as advocated and defended by classical liberals such as Mill (1859) and Feinberg (1973, 1884, 1986). However, their interest is in the legitimate limits of state power, rather than the moral obligations of non-maleficence and beneficence as such, although there is clearly a relation between the legal and moral considerations. They suggest that an individual's liberty may be legitimately restricted by other parties when the proposed action is likely to cause harm to other individuals. A distinction is made between an act performed with the intention of intervening in the life of another individual to prevent harm to that individual, and where the same act is intended to prevent harm to third parties. The former may be a form of paternalism (and therefore wrong) whereas the latter act may be justified through the application of the harm to others principle (and therefore justifiable). The focus in this chapter, as suggested earlier, is upon our moral obligations relating to 'harm to others' considerations rather than the legal obligations that concerned Mill and Feinberg. In the next section I will explore how HOP can be related to the issue of our moral obligations in relation to vaccinations.

sometimes take precedence. Others, drawing on the traditional distinction between perfect and imperfect duties, might want to suggest that non-maleficence will generally (or always?) take precedence over beneficence.

[13] My own sympathies are with Frankena rather than Beauchamp and Childress on this issue.

[14] Indeed, at least in relation to some diseases, the potential harm may be so great as to justify legal compulsion for such vaccinations. However, in this chapter I'm only concerned with an individual's moral obligation to be vaccinated. Discussion of any such legal obligations must be left for another occasion.

10.3. The Harm to Others Argument and Vaccinations

So how might the HOP apply in the context of a general argument about vaccinations for contagious diseases? An argument can be constructed as follows:

1. Contagious diseases that might result in (more than trivial) harm can be passed on to others through non-intentional action.
2. Such a risk of harm can be reduced through vaccination of any potential source individual in advance (where a relevant vaccine exists).
3. We have a general moral obligation not to cause harm to others through our own actions and inactions.
4. Given 1 and 2, an individual can reduce the risk of causing (non-trivial) harm to others through vaccination for (serious) contagious disease.

Conclusion: Given 3 and 4, we are morally obligated to have vaccinations for (serious) contagious diseases (where available).

I'm assuming that advocates of HOP (whether appealing to non-maleficence or beneficence) are likely to support such an argument because the refusal of a vaccination for a serious contagious disease is likely to increase the risk of harm to others who have not voluntarily put themselves at such risk. By this I mean that, on this view, there may be no obligation upon an individual arising from HOP where the harm caused to those individuals affected has arisen because *they* decided not to be vaccinated. However, not all individuals potentially affected by contagious diseases fall into this category because a significant number of individuals are potential victims of the disease and therefore at increased risk of harm even though this is not as a result of their voluntary decision to run that risk. Therefore, it can be argued, by failing to vaccinate yourself against a contagious disease such as diphtheria or polio where an effective agent exists it is not just your own health that you put at risk through your inaction. This means that a decision not to vaccinate in such circumstances is not like a failure to consent to a blood transfusion where you are the only individual directly affected. In the vaccination situation your action raises the risk of harm to 'innocent' others and it might therefore be argued that HOP applies and that you are therefore obligated to be vaccinated for the relevant diseases as a reasonable measure to prevent such potential harm. The situation of non-vaccination in relation to contagious diseases can be contrasted with a decision not to be vaccinated for tetanus. Here the decision has no implications for any third parties. Any (fully informed) non-vaccinated individual affected by the disease has only put themselves at risk of such a harm and must then accept the consequences of their actions when harm occurs (if it does).

However, there are a number of possible grounds for suggesting that HOP should not be applied in this type of case. The first is that it might be argued that HOP should only apply in cases where harm (or risk of harm) is intentionally created. It could be that this is not the case here, as it was never intended that the affected party should be harmed even if the failure to vaccinate was intentional. However it is not clear this will work as the same argument could be mounted in other potential situations where we might expect HOP to be applied. For example, it would seem reasonable to apply HOP in a situation where I intentionally run some risk of causing you harm, but do not intend to cause such harm, such as if I am increasing the risk of fire in my house due to my hobbies (e.g. creating metal sculptures) and your house is attached to mine. I do not intend to cause you harm, but you are at greater risk of harm as a result of my actions. It can then be argued that I am under an obligation to take reasonable precautions to prevent such foreseeable harm. In the case of vaccine-preventable contagious diseases a strong case can be made for such vaccinations counting as a reasonable way to prevent non-intended harm (especially if the disease is likely to cause serious harm or death and the vaccine is effective). HOP may, therefore, impose an obligation to reduce the risk of harm as well as not to cause harm to others.[15]

The second possible grounds for arguing that HOP cannot apply in this case is to argue more directly that the potential risk of any serious harm resulting from any individual's inaction in relation to decisions about vaccination is just too small (or perhaps too remote) to count as significant enough for HOP to apply. However, it might be responded that it is the case that certain types of contagious disease are very harmful (indeed potentially deadly) and that even if there is just a small risk of harm resulting from

[15] There may be other reasons to accept the importance of taking account of the agent's contributions towards increasing a non-intentional risk of harm. One example would be where an individual was infected with a disease whilst on holiday or a business trip after failing to obtain an available vaccination before their trip, and upon return, they then non-intentionally pass on the disease to non-vaccinated individuals in their home country. In such a case, where the risk of infection abroad is known beforehand and an effective vaccine is available, HOP is likely to apply. See Verweij (2005) and Dawson (forthcoming) for discussion.

your actions or inactions this is enough to mean that it is reasonable to hold that HOP applies (especially if the action to be taken by you to attain this end is minor with only a small risk of harm as a result of side-effects). It is generally the case that although certain types of risk are highly remote they are so significant if they do occur that we take great care to ensure that they are unlikely. For example, although the risk of harm from flying in an aeroplane is low, mechanisms and procedures are in place to try and ensure that such risks are as low as possible. If I can reduce such other-related risks of harm, and the costs are not too great to me as an individual, it seems reasonable to argue that I am obligated to do so.

The third possible objection is to suggest that the distinction between acts and omissions is morally relevant here.[16] The idea might be that HOP only applies to the consequences of actions and not omissions. However, such a response does not seem plausible as harm to others can clearly and directly follow as a result of all sorts of omissions. If you travel on a railway where maintenance has not been performed you are at increased risk of harm as a result of an omission. The railway company cannot plausibly rely upon the acts/omission distinction as a defence when harm is caused. On this view, the principle will apply in cases of omission where harm to others is reasonably foreseeable as a result of an omission. This is certainly true in both the case of railway maintenance and that of a failure to vaccinate; both omissions foreseeably increase the risk of harm to others.

Let's assume, then, that HOP can be applied in the vaccination for contagious diseases scenario. We can now consider what difference it might make to the argument whether herd protection exists in a population or not. Where herd protection does not exist it might be argued that no harm to others comes about as a result of *my* omission to vaccinate because whilst such a decision adds to the non-vaccinated population it is not the decisive act that created the non-existence of herd protection. This, of course, is true. On the other hand, the lower the number of participants in any vaccination programme the further we are from herd protection and therefore my omission does contribute to the raising of the risk of harm to others even if it is in an infinitely small way.[17] Whilst HOP suggests we have a general obligation

---

[16] See Dare (1998) for discussion of acts/omissions in relation to vaccinations.

[17] Of course, it might be argued that even after herd protection is attained an individual's failure to vaccinate will increase the risk of them causing harm to others. This is true. However,

to not bring about harm to others as a result of our actions, I have argued that it can also be used to imply that where we can perform an action to reduce the risk of foreseen harm to others through undergoing vaccination (at least where herd protection does not exist) then we may be obligated to do so.

10.4. The Existence of Herd Protection and the No Additional Benefit Argument

If the argument above is sound, individuals may be under a moral obligation to vaccinate themselves to ensure that others are not put at increased risk of harm due to their omission (at least where herd protection does not exist). By contrast it is hard to see how harm to others considerations can be used to justify an obligation to vaccinate where herd protection does already exist precisely because there will, on the whole, be no additional risk of harm to third parties created by my individual decision not to be vaccinated where herd protection already exists.[18] This point can be made through considering an argument that I will call the 'no additional benefit' argument (NAB). It appeals to the idea of herd protection being a public good as it is vital to the argument that the benefits of herd protection are nonexcludable. The argument depends upon the fact that there is a possibility of opting out of contributing to something where you will already gain a share of the benefits due to the actions of others; in this case the existence of herd protection. As suggested before all individuals in the relevant population benefit from the existence of herd protection including those that have not been vaccinated—whether through a choice to opt-out or due to circumstances beyond their control (such as an allergy to one or more component of a vaccine, etc.). NAB strengthens the argument against an obligation to vaccinate where herd protection already exists by pointing out that there is not only no additional benefit to others in you being vaccinated, but there

the chance of any individual contributing to such harm is much greater where herd protection does not exist because once herd protection exists the risk of epidemics falls dramatically.

[18] This is subject to at least two possible exceptions. The first is if, for some reason, I deliberately set out to infect those that I know to be vulnerable to infection because they are not vaccinated. The second is to do with the negligent but non-intentional introduction of a disease to a community from abroad. See also note 20 below.

is, in addition, a potential cost to you, as an individual, in undergoing such a vaccination if there is *any* possibility of side-effects from the vaccination. Whilst it might be considered rational to protect yourself through vaccination, given the balance of such risks, NAB suggests that it does not seem reasonable to argue that you are morally obligated to undergo vaccination (where herd protection exists in a population and you choose not to be vaccinated).

The no additional benefit argument (NAB) can be sketched as follows:

1. One important benefit of vaccination programmes is only felt where an adequate number of the population are vaccinated so that herd protection is established.

2. There can be no obligation upon an individual to run any risk of harm associated with an action where there is no additional benefit to be derived from that action.

3. There is no additional benefit (to reduce harm to others) to be brought about by vaccination where herd protection exists within a population.

4. In addition, once herd protection is achieved, any potential risk of harm caused by the vaccination to the vaccinated individual is run without any gain in benefit to others.

Conclusion: Given these premises there is a strong argument to say that in such circumstances there is no moral obligation to be vaccinated.

Many people will have some intuitive sympathy with NAB. However, it might be given some additional theoretical support through an appeal to consequentialist reasoning. The benefits of seeking to ensure herd protection are great. Indeed as argued before, such a result secures an important public good. However, once herd protection is achieved in the relevant population it is not clear that the idea of a moral obligation to be vaccinated makes sense. Such a position might be supported via two possible consequentialist justifications: the first one a practical one and the second one based on the idea of harm reduction. The first or practical response might be to argue that although such a position strictly produces an injustice, in that not all are subjected to the same potential harms, it is not worth the effort of pursuing any kind of enforcement just to obtain equality in relation to such risks, given the fact that the public good already exists. The second argument based on harm reduction is perhaps stronger and argues that it would be wrong to pursue higher rates of vaccination if there is *any* chance of harm from vaccinations given that herd protection already exists (and such vaccinations are not necessary to reduce harm to others as discussed above). Indeed, it can be argued that the harms-benefits profile of vaccination shifts in such circumstances, and that it becomes unethical to condemn any one refusing to be vaccinated in such circumstances.

Of course there will still be strong pragmatic reasons in favour of seeking to aim at or to maintain vaccination rates at as high a rate as possible within any population, even if levels are currently sufficient to ensure theoretical herd protection. This is for two main reasons. Firstly, because there will always be a small but significant group that have not been (or cannot be) vaccinated even if they (or their parents, where we are talking of young children) wish to do so. Secondly, allowance must be made for the fact that it is immensely difficult to attain and then maintain herd protection levels in any population given the effort this requires from so many different individuals. This difficulty will be increased if as is the case in most countries in the world the population is subject to incoming and outgoing movement through travel and migration. As a result of these two reasons the number of intentionally non-vaccinated individuals that can be carried by any population without thereby threatening herd protection will be smaller than might be otherwise thought. In general, the higher the level of immunity in any population, the better. Therefore, anyone interested in establishing herd protection should aim for one hundred percent coverage of the population, knowing that in reality this can never be achieved.

In conclusion then it looks as though HOP can be used to generate an other-regarding moral obligation for vaccination for at least some contagious diseases where herd protection does not exist because of the possible increase in harm brought about through my omission. However, where herd protection does exist there is no extra risk of harm produced through my omission. What this suggests is that anyone wishing to argue in favour of an obligation to vaccinate where herd protection does exist needs more than HOP to succeed. One possibility is some appeal to the idea of strict mutuality of obligation and I will consider such an argument in the next section.

10.5. NAB as a Free-Rider Argument

The idea of strict mutuality of obligation provides the possibility of a more principled objection to NAB based on the thought that we can construct a type of 'free-rider' argument in relation to vaccinations.[19] Such arguments suggest that where individuals derive benefits from participation in a society, group or population, justice requires that they should contribute a fair share of the effort or risks that it might be necessary to run to achieve that benefit.[20] We can characterise the free-rider argument in relation to vaccination as an argument that whilst herd protection may be a public good we should not ignore the fact that herd protection is a nonexcludable and indivisible public good when we are thinking about our obligations in this area. On this view we should all be obligated to contribute to that good (whether or not we really need to do so to actually create herd protection). Such a view might be defended on two separate grounds. The first derives from the work of Hart (1955) and focuses on mutually binding obligations. The second from Kant (1788) focuses on the mutual obligations that follow from membership of a moral community.

Hart's principle of mutual restriction states that: 'when a number of persons conduct any joint enterprise according to rules and thus restrict their liberty, those who have submitted to these restrictions when required have a right to a similar submission from those who have benefited from submission' (1955: 185). Hart's interest in his paper is in the nature of political obligation, rather than the nature of moral obligations. However, his discussion can be used by way of analogy to sketch an account of moral obligations that many will find attractive. On this view, anyone deriving a benefit from the actions of a group is morally required to perform the same action. Enjoying a shared benefit requires sharing any potential costs. In the vaccination case, once the public good of herd protection exists, everyone benefits from its existence; therefore all are obligated to contribute in the same equal way, by undergoing vaccination for the relevant disease.

---

[19] Of course the assumptions behind free-rider arguments might be questioned. For example, it might be argued that it is not obvious that people are motivated by self-interest on all occasions, nor that the existing empirical evidence supports the existence of free-rider situations in the real world. See Asch and Gigliotti (1991) for discussion of these points.

[20] However, it is possible to argue that the application of straightforward free-rider arguments is less plausible in the vaccination case than, say, in the application of a parallel argument to the issue of paying taxes. This is because there are clear risks to the participating individual in the vaccination case (from side-effects of the vaccine) which are not apparent in the taxation case. This may make a significant difference to any judgments about risks and benefits.

This is not because this is the best way to maintain the good of herd protection (a consequentialist reason), but because it is considered morally important to act towards others in the same way they have acted in the past where you have benefited from their actions (a mutuality reason). The important point is that this view suggests that we owe this to others purely on the basis of having a share in the benefit whether or not we have consented or agreed to it beforehand. Whilst we might object to having to contribute in this way, even so, we cannot side-step our obligation to participate.[21]

It is also possible to construct a Kantian argument with similar results.[22] Here the emphasis will be upon the idea that the maxim that I propose as a guide for action must be able to be universalisable. If I propose, 'I'll opt out, whilst taking the benefit' as a possible maxim, this is clearly not universalisable as it will undermine the existence of herd protection. Kant's categorical imperative (1788) commits anyone adopting his views to think about individual action as having implications for the whole community or population. If my proposed action cannot be universalised then it cannot be a moral action. Kant explicitly emphasises the community aspect to moral obligation in the so-called third formulation of the categorical imperative and his talk of a 'kingdom of ends'.

Both the Hartian and Kantian accounts suggest that we may be morally required to perform a certain action even though it is not clear that anyone will benefit, because on such a view moral rightness is not determined by considerations relating to benefit. In general, many will support such a

---

[21] A similar argument is used by Rawls (1971: 267–8) to suggest that everyone will need to be bound by the rules of a state to ensure that no one is disadvantaged. Nozick (1974) argues against such a view when he suggests that it is wrong for any individual to be bound into an obligation unless he or she has individually consented to such an obligation. Again, we need to take care as this discussion relates to political obligation. However, we can consider a parallel moral case and consider whether such a Nozickian view would ignore the fact that such things as herd protection are nonexcludable public goods. This might mean that individual consent is less important in such a context because not all beneficiaries need to agree in advance to the construction of the good from which even non-contributory members will benefit. See also Arneson (1982) for discussion of public goods and justice considerations.

[22] However, note that Kant seems to be critical of smallpox vaccination as he holds it is potentially interfering with a duty to self. See Kant (1797: 6, 424). I owe this point to Harry Lesser.

view, even if they are troubled by the implication that there is therefore an obligation to undergo vaccination. However, both these accounts can be opposed on the basis that it does not really seem right that individuals should be exposed to an unnecessary risk of harm for the sake of such a formal justice or mutuality requirement. Many people's intuitions will be that there is something wrong here. The basis of this disquiet might well be the idea that some things including risks of harms are just not the types of things that are subject to the requirement for just distribution across all those who benefit in this particular way. The argument might go that otherwise implausible parallel cases would also be justifiable, such as an argument that the risk of radiation damage should also be equalised through a distribution of an appropriate amount of radioactive materials to all households. This just seems absurd. One reasonable conclusion from this discussion is the thought that the benefits consequent upon action are vital to our judgment about our moral obligations in relation to harm to others.[23]

Another possible argument against the free-rider point is to appeal once again to HOP, as outlined above, to argue that where herd protection already exists it appears unreasonable to suggest that any harm will occur to third parties as a result of my inaction. This means that HOP does not apply. Indeed, the only likely risk of harm is to the individual themselves (through the actual vaccination and any possible side-effects) and in such circumstances it is for the individual to refuse vaccination if they so wish through an appeal to a respect for their autonomy coupled with the thought that such a consideration clearly takes priority in circumstances where the harm-to-others issue does not arise. Of course an individual might voluntarily undertake the vaccination within the context of a population where herd protection exists, but I have been exploring what moral obligations might fall upon the competent individual wishing to opt out of a vaccination programme.

The discussion in this section therefore suggests that NAB survives as an argument. It can be supported by consequentialist reasoning through

---

[23] Of course, this is not meant to be an argument against mutual obligations or the categorical imperative as such, just a suggestion that these two approaches are two possible ways to try and avoid a free-rider argument in this context.

an appeal to likely harms and benefits, and seems immune to formal 'mutuality' or 'justice' considerations. We may have obligations to the members of a group, of which we are part, but such obligations are not necessarily obligations that impose the need for mutual action where there is no benefit (to the other members of the group) and some risk (to the individual). I must take into account the consequences for others of my actions and omissions but I am not committed to performing a particular act just because others have performed the same act previously (even when I gain the benefit from their previous actions). Indeed, as mentioned previously, given the shift in the harm-benefits profile of the action, it might be argued that to suggest that an individual is morally obligated to perform an action where no third party will benefit is in turn morally wrong. Herd protection is indeed an important public good. However, whilst no one should do anything to undermine it, we are not morally obligated (at least on liberal grounds) to contribute towards it (where it already exists) even when we may enjoy the benefits.

10.6. Conclusions

The securing of the public good of herd protection can be considered to be so important that it justifies a moral obligation to undergo vaccination for at least some contagious diseases. Where herd protection does not exist harm to others considerations can be used to justify an obligation to be vaccinated (as a contribution to reducing risk of harm in the population). However, in most cases where herd protection already exists such a moral obligation can not be justified by appeal to harm to others or free-rider arguments. In such a situation the no additional benefit argument justifies an opt-out from vaccination by an individual when they wish to invoke it. However, individuals are of course free to participate in such a vaccination programme, if they wish, even when herd protection exists. Indeed, although in this chapter I've been exploring whether there are any principled reasons in favour of a moral obligation to receive a vaccination even when an individual wishes to opt out, we should also be aware that there are strong pragmatic reasons for encouraging vaccinations even when herd protection for a particular disease exists in a population.[24] Herd protection is such an important public good that whilst in some circumstances it might be argued that we are not formally morally obligated to act to uphold it, we should act as if we were.

---

[24] There may well be other moral arguments in favour of such obligations, but in this chapter I'm exploring the obligations that might arise within a traditional liberal framework.

11

Tobacco Discouragement: A Non-Paternalistic Argument

Marcel Verweij[1]

11.1. Introduction

Suppose that academic philosophers are often unhappy persons. On the one hand, they love to think systematically, to teach and to write philosophical papers. On the other, their knowledge of human predicaments makes them more sad than other people. Moreover, the number of academic positions is limited. Some colleagues are very successful and famous, but most philosophers just have a difficult life with limited success. Suppose I think it is better for you to start a career as, say, a waiter in a restaurant. We have discussed this before. Though you agree that a career as a waiter might be enjoyable and probably more successful than a teaching job in philosophy, you still want to be, and to stay, an academic philosopher. Now I can try to improve your life by making it more difficult to practice philosophy and more attractive to become a waiter. If this policy would be successful, that is, if you started to dislike your life as a philosopher so much that you preferred to change your

[1] While developing my arguments I have benefited from discussions with numerous colleagues, notably Bruce Jennings, Angus Dawson, Frans Brom, Richard Ashcroft, and Mariëtte van den Hoven. I am also grateful for the discussion with participants at a Society of Applied Philosophy workshop 'Public Health, Ethical Theory and Public Goods' in Gonville and Caius College, Cambridge, in July 2004.

life and indeed became a waiter, then you would probably be much better off. You would have left behind the hard-to-fulfil desires that most philosophers have (to teach in Cambridge, for example). Instead you will probably have the much easier-to-satisfy desires that most waiters have. How to do this? Well, let's first inform you about the pleasures of being a waiter, and we can emphasise the difficulties philosophers have to deal with. We can raise the salaries of waiters and reduce your salary. It would also be very helpful to reduce the number of academic journals, and hence, reduce the possibilities of you having your papers published. Simultaneously, we'll offer courses that support you in your choice to change your career. The more pervasive this philosophy discouragement policy is, the greater its chances of success.

Yet I expect that many of us would call such a policy unjustifiably paternalistic, especially because it is aims to change *your* preferences for *your own* good. A pervasive policy that aims to affect your preferences and possibilities to do philosophy in many different ways seems manipulative rather than persuasive.

The fact that there are very many unhappy philosophers that can be 'helped' in this way, and that a *public* policy like this could also change the mind of young persons who are still considering the unfortunate choice to study philosophy, will, I think not rebut this charge of unjustified paternalism. Such a 'public' philosophy discouragement policy would be as paternalistic as the individual policy, as it seems to involve some manipulation rather than persuasion. Moreover, we might be especially sceptic of a government that aims to affect people's preferences in such a way. Hence, the policy is certainly not made more justifiable (or less paternalistic) if it is applied more general, yielding the same benefits—through the same means—for more people.

This chapter is not about unhappy philosophers, but about unhealthy tobacco use. The harmful effects of smoking for the smokers themselves, and for people who inhale second hand smoke, are real. Tobacco policies aim to protect third parties from smoke, and such policies might find sufficient support in the harm principle. Yet tobacco policies also aim *to discourage people from smoking*. I will mostly ignore the former policies, and focus on tobacco discouragement. My main problem is that these latter policies are vulnerable to the same anti-paternalist critique as my fictitious philosophy-discouragement policy. In order to resolve this problem, I'll argue that tobacco discouragement is a public good, and that the benefits of such a policy exceed the health benefits of individual smokers.

11.2. Tobacco Discouragement: Changing People's Preferences

Like most other countries, the Netherlands has implemented a number of measures that aim to discourage people to smoke.[2] Tobacco advertisements are prohibited; smoking is not allowed in many public and many semi-public places; employees have a right to a 'smoke-free' working place, which has motivated controversial smoking prohibitions in nursing homes and psychiatric hospitals, and which is motivating a planned ban on smoking in pubs and restaurants. Moreover, the places where tobacco products are sold are limited; taxes on tobacco are high; it is forbidden to sell tobacco products to young persons (<16 years); training programmes are offered for people who want to stop smoking and of course there are a lot of 'commercials' that either emphasise the risks of smoking, or, more recently, that simply indicate that it is 'cool' to refrain from smoking.

Evidently, if the number of smokers would strongly decrease in the next ten years, this would count as a success. After all, smoking is one of the most prominent threats to our highly valued health. Tobacco use is a major cause of lung cancer, ischemic heart disease and chronic airways obstruction. The US Centers for Disease Control estimated that, during 1995–1999, smoking caused 440,000 premature deaths each year in the United States.[3]

The general message that smoking compromises health is well known and publicly communicated time and again, but, apparently, people continue to smoke or start smoking. One factor is that many heavy cigarette smokers are addicted to nicotine and therefore have been unsuccessful in their attempts to quit smoking. Another important factor is that many persons simply do not care enough about the risks, or they accept the possibility that their smoking behaviour might lead to disease and premature death.

Tobacco discouragement policies aim to change these attitudes. They focus on people's behaviour, their wants and preferences and their strength

[2] By 'tobacco discouragement policies' I mean policies that aim to reduce the number of smokers through changing their behaviour. For example, government bodies and health professionals may discourage the use of tobacco through information campaigns, empowerment, or a reduction in the opportunities to buy and use tobacco, or eventually to prohibit smoking. A prohibition is often not seen as a form of tobacco discouragement, but as a measure to protect third parties against passive smoking.

[3] *Morbidity and Mortality Weekly Report* (2002), 51(14): 300–3.

to live according to 'non-smoking' preferences and withstand temptations to smoke. The aim is that smokers will resist, reject or downplay their smoking preferences, and that non-smokers will refrain from adopting a desire to start smoking. To aim at attempting to get people to reject some of their actual or existing wants and desires is controversial.[4] After all, in a democratic society, government should take people seriously, and this involves taking their attitudes, values, and preferences seriously. In short, policies that aim to change people's attitudes require a very strong justification. Moreover, tobacco discouragement goes beyond rational persuasion. The comprehensiveness and pervasiveness of various interventions and programmes in different areas of life (including mass media communication, prominent warnings on products, constraints on possibilities to purchase and smoke tobacco, tax policies, etc.) suggest that they are somewhat manipulative and not simply persuasive in nature.

For these reasons, it is far from self-evident that tobacco discouragement policies are morally justified, even if these policies are effective in reducing tobacco use, and, consequently, in reducing tobacco related morbidity and mortality. After all, the smoking related morbidity and mortality among smokers can be seen as a consequence of their own choices and preferences. Policies that aim to change a person's preferences for the sake of her own health are strongly paternalistic and therefore difficult to justify. If the benefits of tobacco policies are simply equivalent to the benefits for discouraged smokers themselves, tobacco discouragement policies is open to criticism for its paternalist character. Paternalist interventions might be justified in special circumstances, for example when nicotine addiction renders smokers' choices substantially non-voluntary. This will certainly hold for many heavy smokers. Yet it will be difficult to uphold such a claim in general, and to

---

[4] Such policy aims raise problems in a pluralistic democratic society, because they presume a strong version of, what Brian Barry (1965: 38ff) calls, ideal-regarding considerations. A liberal policy would be based on want-regarding principles. These principles start from the wants that people in society actually have, and evaluate policies by evaluating their effects on want-satisfaction. (This may involve both a focus on aggregate want-satisfaction, as in utilitarianism, and a focus on the distribution of opportunities people have to satisfy their wants). Ideal-regarding considerations diverge from the given wants of people. A modest ideal-regarding approach is to take people's wants as a starting point for policy, yet to presume other rankings among a person's wants than those of the person himself or herself. A step further would be to exclude certain wants from consideration. An ideal-regarding principle in the strongest sense would take into account considerations that are independent from the actual wants of persons.

argue that all smoking preferences are non-voluntary, and that therefore paternalist interventions aimed at changing these attitudes might be universally justified. I will discuss the topic of addiction and voluntariness several times, but my route for avoiding anti-paternalist critique will be different.

The charge of unjustified paternalism might also be avoided if public health programmes emphasise that there are also *public* concerns at issue, for example by explaining that effective tobacco discouragement is not just for the benefit of smokers, but that it also serves a public interest or public good.

11.3. Harm to Others

The strongest argument about tobacco policies in a democratic pluralist society concerns the fact that tobacco products cause harm. Protecting people from being harmed by others, is one of the primary concerns in a liberal society and in contractarian justifications in political and ethical theory. This is indeed a public concern, as it applies to every member of the public, and every member of the public benefits from the security that is created by harm-preventing policies. The harm principle is a very strong claim which may be invoked (and is even meant to be invoked in order) to justify imposing restrictions on individual liberty (Mill 1859; Feinberg 1984).

The harm principle can be relevant for various elements in tobacco policies. 'Second hand' smoke can be harmful for non-smokers, therefore interventions that set limits to smoking practices in order to prevent passive smoking might find support in the harm principle. The principle is however not directly relevant for tobacco discouragement policies. Before discussing these issues, I turn to a possible application of the harm principle that might be more basic.

11.3.1. A Ban on Sale

The harm principle might not only apply to the behaviour of smokers, but also to the actions of tobacco companies and retailers. These organizations are marketing and selling products that are both harmful and addictive. Arguably, if a company would now develop a new consumer product with similar harmful and addictive characteristics, relevant government bodies such as the US Food and Drug Administration would have a strong case for deciding not to accept it in the free market. One might see an analogy in the way drugs like heroin or cocaine are treated. Some drugs that are banned in many countries are less addictive and harmful than tobacco is. A ban on drugs, backed up by fierce sanctions, should not be just seen as a paternalist intervention towards drug abusers, but more importantly, as criminal prosecution of producers and sellers. Hence, the radical way to 'discourage' use of tobacco would be to prohibit the sale of tobacco altogether. Such measures have been proposed before, and they might possibly be supported by appeal to the harm principle.[5] Obviously, a ban on tobacco products would raise numerous problems, as smoking has been an accepted practice for centuries. It will be very difficult to ban this practice, and national prohibitions could be futile if cigarettes remain available abroad.

However, there is also a preliminary question to be answered. Is the claim that smokers are harmed by tobacco companies' offer of harmful products justified? From a liberal perspective one might argue that if persons voluntarily accept the risks of the products they purchase, the retailer or producer cannot be blamed that they sell harmful products. *Volenti non fit injura*: there is no harm (in the moral or legal sense) if persons deliberately and voluntarily engage in risky behaviour. In such a case, they cannot be the victim of harmful practices of the tobacco industry or the retailers. In other words, if smokers can be held sufficiently responsible for their purchase of tobacco products and smoking behaviour, the harm principle would not provide a basis for prohibiting the sale of tobacco.

Now many smokers are addicted to nicotine and have little success in their attempts to quit smoking. Nicotine addiction might therefore render smoking a non-voluntary (or at least insufficiently voluntary) act.[6] This premise provides support for the application of the harm principle—or more precise, it implies that the volenti reply does not hold. It is not completely clear to what extent the premise about non-voluntariness is valid. Current practices and policies—at least in the Netherlands—seem to assume that adult smokers are sufficiently responsible: a ban on tobacco is

---

[5] Robert Goodin (1989) argues that there might be a case for a prohibition of over-the-counter sale of cigarettes.

[6] Although I now focus on interventions that put restrictions on sale in a free market—hence interventions that limit the freedom of tobacco sellers and producers—this premise would also support a *paternalist* policy towards the smokers themselves.

not a prominent theme in political debate; and notwithstanding numerous tobacco discouragement measures, stopping smoking is considered the responsibility of each individual herself.[7] In this chapter I will not attempt to answer the question whether nicotine addiction necessarily implies that smoking is to be considered non-voluntary—even though this issue will come back at several stages of my analysis. For now it is enough to conclude that the harm principle might support a ban on the sale of cigarettes, but that this argument hinges on the premise that smoking is not sufficiently voluntary. This chapter will however focus on public justification for tobacco discouragement and not on tobacco prohibition.

11.3.2. Preventing Passive Smoking

The risks of passive smoking are more common ground for appealing to the harm principle. The US Center for Disease Control estimated that approximately 35,000 of the earlier mentioned 440,000 annual tobacco deaths are due to the effects of 'second hand smoke'. Hence there are strong reasons to protect non-smokers from the risk imposed on them by smokers. Most Western countries are imposing more and more restrictions on smoking in public places and semi-public places (e.g. pubs, workplaces, sports facilities, etc.) The harm principle offers sufficient support for implementing smoking prohibitions in places where non-smokers will be harmed by 'second hand smoke'.

Yet, again, the aim of preventing harm to others is different from the aim of discouraging people from smoking. The harm principle supports policies that protect people from harm imposed by companies or other persons, but it does not support protecting persons against their own unhealthy behaviour. At least not in a direct way.

There could be an indirect way in which the aim to protect persons against harm imposed by others may support tobacco discouragement policies. The health problems of passive smoking will probably be most salient in families with actively smoking parents. Small children may be more vulnerable to the harmful effects of passive smoking than grown-ups. If heavy smoking by parents imposes serious health risks on children, this could be a reason to

---

[7] This latter statement has been explicitly mentioned as an argument against a proposal to cover nicotine replacement therapies in the Dutch basic health insurance package. Tweede Kamer der Staten-Generaal (2000), TK 30–2628, 30 November.

protect these children against their parents' harmful behaviour. Moreover, living in a smoker's environment will facilitate, if not stimulate, children to start smoking themselves. In a recent report on the effects of passive smoking, the Dutch Health Council pointed out that passive smoking at home remains outside the scope of restrictive tobacco policies (Health Council of the Netherlands 2003). Yet, the harm principle might give support to government interference with the smoking behaviour of parents. Such a policy however will face serious drawbacks.

First, it involves interference in the private sphere of parents and their families. On a theoretical level, such interventions may be justified, as the focus of the harm principle is precisely to set limits to personal freedom and privacy. In a way, the boundaries between the public sphere and the private sphere are drawn by considerations like the harm principle: child abuse can not be considered immune from public interference if it occurs in a private sphere, because protection against harm is a public matter. For a strong justification however it is not sufficient to recognise that the harm principle is relevant. Interfering between parents and children may have harmful effects on their relationship (and hence on the children and parents themselves) as well. Therefore, the dangers for children should also be clear and concrete in order to give the considerations of protecting against harm enough strength to outweigh countervailing arguments. And this point may be questioned: the harmful effects of passive smoking will only occur over a long period in which the child is exposed to smoke.[8] There is not a single act of the smoking parent that poses a serious threat: the harm is not in one assignable act but in the habit of the parent. This also gives rise to other, more pragmatic reasons for foregoing restrictions for smoking in the private sphere. A prohibition upon smoking in the neighbourhood of children would be impractical and unenforceable unless the private sphere would be opened up completely.

Yet the goal of protecting children from the harmful effects of their parents' smoke may be aimed at in a less drastic and direct way. If one concludes that it is difficult to justify interference in the family, the best way to prevent harm might be to discourage parents to smoke. Midwives will normally warn pregnant women that smoking will harm their child. The Dutch Health Council recommends including frequent warnings about passive smoking

[8] Harm might be more direct and short-term in some cases, e.g., smoking during pregnancy might negatively affect the growth and health of the foetus, hence cause harm to the future child.

in the standard job description of individuals working in child health care. In 1998, the Netherlands Organization for Information about Tobacco Risks also started a large campaign 'Smoking? Not if the child is in the neighbourhood'. In an animated cartoon, the father of a new-born baby forbids the grandfather to enter the house with a cigar. Obviously, it is not so much the grandparents of the baby, but the parents themselves who are addressed by this cartoon. The occasional cigar of grandfather will be far less harmful than the frequent cigarettes smoked by the child's mother. The interesting element in this campaign is its explicit moralistic nature. The message is: it is all right that parents tell others (and, more importantly, tell each other) that it is a bad thing to smoke in the neighbourhood of the children. This moralism[9] is strengthened by the fact that this mass-media campaign aims at a very broad audience: it goes far beyond the private sphere of discussions between health professional and parent. This facilitates the development of attitudes and beliefs (among parents and others) that people have a moral responsibility not to smoke in the neighbourhood of children. Below, I will come back to this feature of health promotion as affecting social norms and not just individual behaviour. For now it is sufficient to conclude that the harm principle may be directly relevant for some elements in a tobacco policy (and support policies that prohibit smoking in public places), but it does not give direct support to tobacco discouragement as such. There is however an indirect way in which the harm principle may plead for tobacco discouragement: in private contexts, the best way to prevent harm to others is to discourage the agents to smoke themselves.

11.4. Economic Costs and Consequentialist Perspectives on Public Health

At first sight the most plausible argument for tobacco discouragement would be consequentialist, where such an approach weighed the aggregate benefits and costs of tobacco policies. If we disregard the direct harmful effects of

[9] The term 'moralism' sometimes has a negative connotation, but this is not what I mean by it. Moralism in the sense of aiming to arouse moral feelings and to stimulate people to adopt and act according to certain moral views may be justified in many contexts. Whether it is justified in this case, or raises ethical problems is, so far, an open question.

smoking on the health of others (after all, such effects can be sufficient for liberty restricting policies), there are still negative consequences for society as a whole. Smoking is a major cause of cancer, cardiovascular and other diseases. Smokers who fall ill will require health care, and in most Western societies the costs of such care are borne by society at large. If these costs are large, then society would have a strong case to discourage smoking, in order to reduce these costs: a weighing of costs and benefits could plea for policies that are successful in reducing the number of people who smoke.[10]

11.4.1. Questionable Premises in the Argument of Costs

However, studies in epidemiology and health economy show that the empirical premises in this argument are questionable. According to Barendregt and colleagues (1997), a major reduction of smoking in society would at first lead to a decrease in health care expenditures, but after a longer period, the costs would increase more substantially. The explanation is well known: the costs of health care are highest in people of old age. Generally, fewer smokers will live to old age than non-smokers do. To put it bluntly, smokers are more likely (than non-smokers) to die before they are struck with the diseases of old age. So crude weighing of financial costs and benefits may not univocally result in arguments for tobacco discouragement policies (Warner 2000).

Such a perspective, focusing on monetary costs and benefits, should however not be considered as decisive in evaluating tobacco policies or more generally, health policies. If these arguments would be decisive, then studies like Barendregt's would count as decisive arguments for encouraging people to start smoking. Moreover, probably many life-saving interventions will generate health care costs in the long run. The basic problem is that this perspective reduces all benefits in monetary terms. This reduction is of course not necessary in a consequentialist perspective. The main benefits of effective tobacco discouragement consist in an increase of disease free life expectancy of people. The value of such effects should not be determined in terms of prevention or the generation of social (health care) expenditures, but primarily by taking into account the value of life and health for all persons involved. Smokers, like non-smokers, will normally prefer a natural healthy

---

[10] The health care costs due to smoking raise problems of justice as well (Wilkinson 1999).

life span above an untimely death. A longer healthy life will give them more opportunities for being happy and seeing their preferences and ideals fulfilled.

11.4.2. A Preference Utilitarian's Perspective

Now, if the value of the smokers' lives for themselves is taken into account, and the pleasures and experiences they will miss due to untimely illness and mortality, it is less clear whether the consequentialist would reject tobacco discouragement.

The most plausible way to take into account the pleasures and experiences of persons themselves and how they themselves value and weigh these pleasures against other pleasures (e.g. smoking), is through a form of preference utilitarianism. Tobacco discouragement policies may be supported from a preference utilitarian perspective if we assume that all persons want to stay healthy and not fall ill and die before they have reached a natural life span. A successful policy could therefore result in an increase of aggregate preference satisfaction; not only preferences regarding health would be better satisfied, but if average life expectancy would rise, people will have more opportunities to see other things in their (longer) life fulfilled. However, this utilitarian strategy raises two questions.

First, tobacco discouragement might indeed promote preference satisfaction, but it does so by seeking to change people's preference sets, or at least by giving less weight to particular desires (viz. desires to enjoy a cigarette). The objective is that people will not develop smoking preferences, will reject smoking preferences or at least give more weight to their preferences for a healthy life. It is not obvious that such a way of promoting preference satisfaction can be justified in a preference-utilitarian theory.[11] Such a theory is problematic if it does not set limits to attempts to *change* people's preferences—which after all are seen as the ultimate appeal for normative reasons. Some constraints on preferences might however be necessary, for example that they be informed or even (in some minimum sense) rational.

The aspect of addiction could then be relevant. If smokers' preferences to smoke are substantially non-voluntary, then there might be good reasons to

---

[11] Possibly, such interventions might be justified in a preference based utilitarian account that focuses on *rational* preferences or otherwise preferences that are well-considered. Still, it is not a priori clear if, in such an account, smoking preferences would always be filtered out.

discount such preferences in a utilitarian calculus. After all, it is difficult to see fulfilment of non-voluntary desires as a good to be promoted. So, if we accept that preferences for smoking are generally non-voluntary, then we might be able to develop a strong utilitarian argument for tobacco discouragement policies. Accepting this premise will however support more drastic anti-tobacco policies as well. In the previous section, I argued that that if smoking preferences and hence choices to buy tobacco products, are substantially non-voluntary, then, combined with the harmful effects of tobacco, this might give strong support to a complete ban on sale of tobacco products.

Now, obviously, stopping smoking is very difficult for most regular smokers. Many see their attempts fail time and again. Many others, however, simply do not want to stop, and others again can and do stop when they try. I have doubts about whether one can safely assume that generally, smoking preferences are sufficiently involuntary or non-autonomous to justify excluding these preferences from utilitarian weighing. The premise that generally, it is very difficult to quit smoking is, I think much easier to accept. Probably, such a premise is too weak to justify discounting of smoking preferences in utilitarian reasoning. In the next section, however, I will argue that this weaker claim, might be very important for justifying tobacco discouragement.

11.4.3. The Need for an Argument in Terms of a Public Good

A second question for the utilitarian argument raises some doubts about the extent to which the utilitarian (preference-based) argument would be sufficient to justify a public policy of tobacco discouragement. In various chapters in this volume it is argued that public health involves more than 'just' the aggregation of private health of all participants. In other words, tobacco discouragement would not just be for the benefit of all discouraged smokers, but there would be external benefits—hence a public good—as well. The argument about costs was indeed a public argument because it focused on external effects of smoking (the effects on health care expenditures; expenditures that must be paid for by all citizens), and not just on the private effects for the smokers themselves. So far, it is not clear why the private preferences and attitudes of persons and the effects of such attitudes on those persons' own health would be a public matter. Hence, even if effective tobacco discouragement policies may lead to a drastic reduction of morbidity and mortality, it is unclear why they should be considered as public health interventions. The utilitarian argument will fail unless it is possible to argue that tobacco discouragement has important benefits that exceed the health benefits of the discouraged members of the target group.

11.5. Tobacco Discouragement as a Public Good

The problem so far is that the two plausible ethical allies of public health, the harm principle and the consequentialist perspective, seem to fall short in supporting tobacco discouragement. The first might support certain prohibitive measures, but it does not support (at least not in a direct way) tobacco discouragement. The utilitarian argument is not completely satisfying as it does not succeed as a public argument for public policy, and it might need assumptions about voluntariness that are too strong to be generally warranted.

In this section I argue that there is another consideration which may be tenable and relevant in a public perspective. I have argued that the utilitarian argument might be problematic as it seems to aim primarily at promoting the private goods of the members of the target group. Many successful public health interventions on the other hand do not, in a direct way, aim at the private health of individuals. They aim at factors affecting the health of large groups of non-assignable persons. Those risk factors are not internal to the biological life and behaviour of those persons; they are part of the physical or social environment of a larger public. Therefore, if some of those risks 'from outside' are reduced, then all will benefit. Infectious diseases control is a good example. Measures that effectively reduce the spread of dangerous viruses increase everyone's chance for a healthy life. Such a reduction can be called a public good in the strict sense: it requires collective action, and the good of protection is non-excludable and indivisible.[12] The benefits are not limited to the persons who participate in the collective action. In other words: the benefits are enjoyed by all regardless as to whether or not they participated in the collective action. Now, can the aims of tobacco discouragement policies, i.e. a situation in which fewer people would smoke than do now, be considered

---

[12] Cf. Chapter 1.

as a public good in this sense? A successful tobacco discouragement policy would result in a reduction in the use of tobacco, hence less people would start smoking and more would stop smoking. The prevalence of smoking would decrease. If this result is to be considered a public good, then it would imply that the benefits are in a way 'open to all' and not just fall to persons who 'participated' in the policy and were discouraged by the policy. In other words, seeing tobacco discouragement as a public good means that the benefits should exceed the benefits experienced by persons who stopped smoking, or who reduced their smoking behaviour, or who decided not to start smoking as a result of the policy. Do such external effects indeed occur in tobacco discouragement? Without saying that smoking is 'contagious', it is obvious that smoking behaviour does have important social determinants. I'll argue that this might help to understand tobacco discouragement as a public good.

11.5.1. Smoking Practices as a Societal Risk Factor

First, whether or not teenagers start smoking will depend to a large extent, on the norms within the groups, families, and communities within which they live. The more one lives among friends and family members who smoke, the more one will think smoking to be normal and uncontroversial, and this will reduce the threshold for starting to smoke as well. So, obviously, the prevalence of smoking in one's environment will be an important determinant for adolescents to start smoking as well. There might even be some pressure of peers, and at least many persons will be eager to follow the example of others. This is not to say that smoking behaviour of teenagers is substantially involuntary or non-autonomous; it is simply a statement about seeing the norms about smoking as an important factor that contributes to a desire to start smoking as well.

Second, many will consider smoking as a social activity, something which is most pleasant and common when one is among others. Moreover, the social component of smoking often has a positive image—at least for smokers. It is not uncommon to hear some people (smokers?) say that generally, it is more pleasant to be among smokers, than among non-smokers. Hence, it is not just that in many contexts, smoking is common, but—despite all warnings about health effects—it is sometimes also given positive value. The group norms about smoking are often reinforced by affirmative images and attitudes.

Third, when one lives among smokers it will be very difficult to stop smoking oneself. Such a context requires a very strong motivation: each time a friend or any other person nearby lights a cigarette an opportunity (hence temptation) arises to ask for a cigarette and start smoking again. Most smokers will find it difficult to stop anyhow, and being in a situation in which lots of others continue to smoke makes the effort of quitting smoking even more difficult.

11.5.2. Tobacco Discouragement as Public Health Intervention

So, to some extent, smoking behaviour is determined by the social context. If tobacco use is common, this will both facilitate (young) persons to start smoking as well as complicate attempts to stop smoking. Again, this is not to endorse some form of social determinism which completely downgrades the role of individual choices. But at least, the social context, notably the attitudes and norms of friends, family, colleagues, etc. towards smoking, is an important contributing factor for one's own attitudes towards smoking. This social context may be considered as a target for public health policies. A reduction in the number of smokers in society, hence a social context in which smoking is less common and evident, makes it easier for smokers to abstain and more easy for not-yet-smokers to refrain from smoking. An important factor that contributes to smoking behaviour would then be weakened. Interventions aiming to reduce the strength of this contributing factor may be considered as analogous to other public health interventions. Many typical public health measures aim to take away risks in the physical and social environment, and in that way, contribute to the health of all living in that environment. In a similar way, tobacco discouragement policies might be considered not just as aiming to improve the health of all smokers, but also, or even primarily, as aiming at creating an environment in which smoking is less common, and in which it will be easier for adolescents not to start smoking and for those who want to stop, to be successful in their efforts. This might be considered as a benefit open to all. Moreover, this context can only be realised through cooperative endeavour. In this way, successful tobacco discouragement could be considered as representing a public good.

This observation might also support the utilitarian argument in the previous section. I concluded that the utilitarian argument would fail as a public argument unless tobacco discouragement yields important benefits that exceed the health benefits of the discouraged members of the target group. In this section I have argued that there are such 'public' benefits.

The observation that tobacco discouragement can be considered as a public good, does not as such imply that such policies might be justified. What policies would be justified would of course depend on the nature of the interventions. Yet the arguments in the previous sections (the indirect application of the harm principle, and the utilitarian line of argument), together with the analysis of tobacco discouragement as a public good, might be sufficient for justifying most common policies.

11.5.3. Are All Common Unhealthy Behaviours 'Public Health' Problems?

There are however a number of problems that arise if my explanation of tobacco discouragement as a public good would be acceptable. First, does not the analysis support much more interventions in the name of public health than we would intuitively consider appropriate? Lifestyle and behaviour are important determinants of health, and smoking is certainly not the only health compromising behaviour that is partly determined by social practices. So, by aiming at the social context as an important factor for individual health compromising behaviour, this argument could open the door to numerous discouragement and encouragement policies regarding food practices, alcohol consumption, occupational contexts, physical exercise, etc. For example, why not focus also on unhealthy food practices and make it more difficult to buy and consume fatty snacks? Why not shutdown all escalators in order to force people to walk up the stairs—hence to promote physical exercise? If all possibilities for health promotion are taken into account, then people's choices and behaviour would be constantly affected and directed by the caring concern of health authorities, and that would seem undesirable (Verweij 1999). Probably this problem can be best answered by pointing at the exceptional character of smoking. It may be doubted whether there are other unhealthy activities that are similarly widespread, similarly guided by social context, similarly risky, and as difficult to abstain from as smoking.

11.5.4. Should a Government Promote or Discourage Particular Views of the Good Life?

Second, and more generally, suppose we accept tobacco discouragement as a public good and have arguments to support the claim that governments should discourage smoking. Is such a claim tenable in the light of the liberal doctrine of neutrality? After all, tobacco discouragement policies seem to promote particular forms of life or conceptions of the good life and discourage others. In a democratic pluralistic society, it can certainly not be justified for a government to promote in a similar way particular religious conceptions of the good life, and discourage others. Can tobacco discouragement be considered as a similar violation of neutrality? For two reasons, I do not think it should be considered as such, but there are some complications.

First, the value that guides tobacco discouragement policies is not a controversial value: it is health. It is not controversial to assume that all persons consider the protection of health to be important. This however is not yet sufficient, because it is far from self-evident that all or most persons would endorse the specific goals of tobacco discouragement, even if they endorse health as a value. In other words many may prefer smoking and accept the risks for their health.

Secondly, even if government should refrain from arguing that persons ought to abstain from smoking in their private lives, government cannot be completely neutral regarding conceptions of a good society. If choices about smoking were completely private and voluntary, then considerations about 'the good society' would be rather irrelevant in this context. However, government should not be neutral if:

1. It is clear that smoking is both addictive and a major cause of mortality;
2. Health is a universal value; and
3. Smoking behaviour is partly determined and sustained by social practices and norms regarding smoking.

It is difficult for individuals to abstain from smoking even if they would like to stop, and it becomes more difficult the more they live in a social context full of opportunities and temptations to light another cigarette. A society in which it is very easy to start smoking but very difficult to refrain from smoking can be considered as undesirable. Even though such a view of society might entail (and promote) particular conceptions of the good life, this should not be a reason to exclude it as a basis for public policy.

11.6. Conclusion

In this chapter I have argued that tobacco discouragement policies are vulnerable to anti-paternalist critique, as far as they aim to affect people's preferences for their own good. Even though most interventions are not coercive, tobacco discouragement might be considered somewhat manipulative given the comprehensive character of the policies. The high mortality and morbidity rates due to smoking seem to suggest an easy utilitarian justification for tobacco discouragement policies, but I have argued the argument is less simple. From a welfarist perspective (and I take preference-utilitarianism as an important form of welfarism), the perspectives and preferences of persons need to be taken seriously, and policies that aim to affect preferences are therefore problematic.

One way to answer the critique is to focus on nicotine addiction, and to argue that smoking preferences and choices can be discounted as they are non-voluntary and non-autonomous. I have expressed some doubts about the correctness of this argument. Yet if this counter-argument is valid, it might yield sufficient reason for a complete ban on tobacco, and policies aiming at tobacco discouragement would seem superfluous.

Another way to answer the critique is to develop an argument that explains how tobacco discouragement might contribute to a public good. This helps to picture tobacco discouragement as a real public health policy—and not just as a paternalist policy aiming to improve the (private) health of many individuals, through changing their own preferences. According to this argument, the ultimate objective of tobacco discouragement is not to change the smokers' desires for their own good, but to affect a current social context that facilitates desires to start smoking and complicates efforts to stop with smoking. Protection against such social determinants of smoking can be considered as a public good for the benefit of all. In this way, tobacco discouragement is not completely different from other public health interventions, such as protection against spread of communicable diseases, environmental policies, or food safety control. Public health interventions are interventions that aim at factors affecting the health of large groups of non-assignable persons. Those risk factors are not internal to the biological life and behaviour of individuals; they are part of the physical or social environment of all. My argument sees smoking practices as an important public risk factor for unhealthy behaviour that is very difficult to refrain from, and tobacco discouragement as a policy that aims to change this social context.

The argument also has implications for responsibility for the health effects of smoking and the availability of support for persons who intend to stop. If the current social environment, in which, given the prevalence of smoking, it is easy to start with, and very difficult to refrain from smoking, is considered as an important factor for smoking behaviour, there is reason for society to assume—to some extent—collective responsibility for smoking practices and tobacco related morbidity. This could be a reason to include therapies and programmes which support smoking cessation (e.g. nicotine replacement therapy) in a public health insurance—at least one can not simply argue that smoking cessation is each person's own responsibility. Moreover, the assumption of collective responsibility makes it less easy to accept that individual smokers who become ill are personally responsible for their illness. Neither can one simply think that tobacco companies carry all of the responsibility for the harms of tobacco. Apparently, with respect to smoking, issues of responsibility are much more complex than that.

12

Informed Consent and the Expansion of Newborn Screening[1]

Niels Nijsingh

The moral acceptability and justifiability of a medical procedure seems partly dependent on whether informed consent has been attained. In many situations it is clear why this is so. There is near consensus that patients should have a say in whether to undergo surgery, particularly if there are alternatives available and when there are clear advantages and disadvantages to the different options. It is generally conceded that patients should be in a position to weigh what is important to them. Furthermore, informed consent is undisputedly an effective way to prevent abuse and exploitation of patients, for example in the context of medical research.[2]

It is tempting to assume that the requirement for informed consent should stretch out over the entire medical domain, so that it would include not only medical research and clinical encounters, but also screening for disease. In this chapter I will look at the requirement for informed consent in

[1] This chapter greatly benefited from the helpful suggestions of Ainsley Newson, Marcus Düwell, Paul Sollie, and Annemarie Kalis. Particular thanks are owed to Marcel Verweij and Angus Dawson for many helpful comments.

[2] However, some, such as Garrard and Dawson (2005) argue that there are limits here.

the practice of newborn screening in the light of technological developments that enable a drastic expansion of the screening program. I will argue that for such an expanded program of newborn screening, informed consent is not an absolute requirement, and even that, on the contrary, *full* informed consent is morally objectionable in this context.

Newborn screening is a practice that takes place in all industrialized countries. The screening itself usually involves the taking of a drop of blood from the heel of a newborn infant. The blood is then analyzed and screened for a variety of inborn diseases (Erbe and Levy 1996).[3] Due to proceeding technological developments it has become possible to screen for an increasing number of diseases and susceptibilities for diseases. Some countries have, in varying degrees, already expanded the screening offer substantially and for other countries drastic expansions are apparently on the way.[4]

For a limited offer, where the benefits are obvious and the harms minimal, the informed consent procedure is generally not a cause for concern. However, expansion might entail that diseases for which screening has less obvious benefits and might even do harm, are added to the program. This raises the question of what the consequences are for the informed consent procedure. It is not obvious that the same considerations hold when the screening program is expanded from one or two diseases to thirty or even more—particularly when the expansions are not uncontroversial.

Some hold that informed consent requirements need to be strengthened as the screening program expands.[5] Some go even further and argue that a thorough informed consent procedure might dissolve some of the initial reservations we might have towards such an expansion. The claim would then be that the informed consent procedure may play a legitimating role, because the more controversial cases are left up to the parents themselves. My goal here is to see what this claim could entail, and to what extent it holds.

---

[3] Interesting ethical comments on the practice of newborn screening that I benefited from in writing this chapter are Ross (2002), Hermerén (1999) and Kerruish and Robertson (2005).

[4] For example, in the Netherlands, the State Secretary of Health recently decided—on recommendation of the Dutch Health Council (Gezondheidsraad 2005)—to expand the current offer of three diseases, to eighteen.

[5] The Dutch Health Council (Gezondheidsraad 2005) and the Nuffield Council of Bioethics (1993) offer good examples, but I dare venture that such a claim is quite regularly implicitly or explicitly endorsed.

12.1. The Expansion of Newborn Screening

Wilson and Jungner (1968) have stated ten criteria for screening, which include that the disease sought for should have an adequate treatment and that it should be an important health problem.[6] The prototypical example in newborn screening programs is phenylketonuria (PKU), which is an early onset mono-factorial disease, where early detection enables one to prevent serious health damage to the child (in particular mental retardation). For decades the criteria of Wilson and Jungner have been widely regarded as minimal requirements for any screening program - and for many countries they still offer a strong guideline for admittance of diseases to the screening program. However, it is now sometimes argued that it may be advisable to screen for untreatable diseases, or very rare diseases, or susceptibilities for disease. I would claim that neither of these categories fit the criteria of Wilson and Jungner.[7] Nevertheless, there may be good reasons to want to include them in the program.[8] These reasons are not just limited to the medical and financial aspects.

A clear example is Duchenne's Muscular Dystrophy (DMD). DMD is an untreatable disease. Patients suffering from DMD will not develop symptoms before they are two or three years old, but from that moment on the disease develops progressively. DMD manifests itself by a degeneration of the muscles. Most DMD patients die in early adulthood. It is a rare, mono-factorial disease.

Although DMD is untreatable, screening for it has some advantages. Not the least of those is that timely diagnosis might prevent the birth of a sibling with the same condition. Furthermore, screening might prevent a long and tiresome diagnostic delay (Mohamed et al. 2000). However, there are clear disadvantages to screening for DMD too. Since the onset of the disease doesn't occur until the third or fourth year of the infant's life, this means

---

[6] See Shickle (1999) for a thorough discussion of the criteria of Wilson and Jungner applied to genetic testing.

[7] It is sometimes argued that 'treatment' should be interpreted more broadly, so as to include decisions about one's mortgage and career. The notion of an 'important health problem' is also a topic of much discussion. I believe that one should be careful not to stretch these notions too far, otherwise there is a danger that they become meaningless.

[8] In fact in some countries screening is performed for untreatable diseases. See Loeber (1999). However, most countries are more hesitant in the implementation of the expanded possibilities.

that parents are confronted with information on a very serious condition that will not become manifest until a few years later. Such information might burden an affected family.

As it turns out, not all parents would like their child to be screened for DMD. Whilst some parents would want to have this sort of information on their child, others indicate that they would not want to know whether their child has DMD (Campbell and Ross 2005; Hosli et al. forthcoming). Both positions seem valid.

At this point one might argue that the desires of the parents are not decisive when considering what is best for the child. One might be tempted to say that the perspective of the parents is irrelevant, because screening is conducted with regard to the interest of the child. The conclusion would then be that the procedure should be made obligatory. I agree that in some instances the decision of the parents may (and should) be overruled (Dawson 2005). I also believe that it is important to distinguish these different perspectives. However, I think that since in the case of (the expansion of) newborn screening it is not obvious that the child's health is at risk when people refuse screening, an obligatory procedure seems hard to justify. This is particularly clear in the case of untreatable diseases, such as DMD, but I think that this argument holds for all diseases for which a possibility to screen exists (Nijsingh forthcoming). There seem to be strong and valid arguments both for *and* against testing for DMD. Given that parents may have good reasons for not participating in a screening program for controversial diseases, they should be able to choose not to. Note that this argument works the other way around too. Given that parents may have good arguments *for* wanting their child tested for DMD, it seems we have an argument for at least giving people the option. I'll return to this point in the concluding section.

DMD is, however, not the only potential expansion that is controversial. There are good reasons—albeit very different ones from those that apply in the case of DMD—for and against screening for extremely rare diseases, for and against screening for susceptibilities, for and against screening for diseases that are less serious and for and against screening for diseases where screening also gives unwanted information, such as carrier status. For each of these diseases a case can be made for and against testing for it, and so offering the option of screening may seem sensible.

Discussions on the desirability of a certain expansion tend to become rather complex (Hosli et al. forthcoming). Quite a few considerations play a role in determining what type of diseases qualify for screening. The resulting complexity is multiplied by the fact that there are a large number of possible expansions that are very different in type and for which as a result a lot of different arguments play a role.

12.2. The Informed Consent Imperative

Informed consent has gradually become ingrained in clinical medical practice. Although the requirement is not completely uncontroversial,[9] there is near consensus that this is an improvement compared to the 'bad old days' of paternalism (Savulescu 1995). However, care for a proper informed consent procedure is less obviously integrated in the practice of screening, which has led to the worry that this infringes the rights of the person subjected to screening. This worry is nicely expressed by Austoker as follows:

'Screening, like most medical interventions, has harms as well as benefits. All the more reason therefore to ensure that patients undergoing screening are fully aware of both the benefits and the harms . . . Failure to obtain truly informed consent for many current preventive interventions is clearly unethical.' (Austoker 1999).

Although in this quote the reference is to screening in general, it seems natural to apply it to the case of newborn screening. As I already mentioned, there *are* harms as well as benefits to newborn screening. It is to be expected that as the screening program expands, there will be more harms, and the benefits will not always be as obvious. Therefore, some argue, if the screening program expands, the informed consent procedure should be improved. It is also sometimes argued that, no matter whether there is an expansion or not, the fact that newborn screening reveals genetic information that might be of a drastic consequence to people's lives, already gives us a reason to set the informed consent standard very high. Let us call the view that stresses the importance of informed consent whenever medical interventions are controversial ('harms as well as benefits'), the Informed Consent Imperative (ICI). The ICI sees an intrinsic link between

---

[9] See O'Neill (2002) for a sharp comment on the current status of and reliance upon informed consent.

the harms and benefits of an intervention and the necessity of informed consent:[10]

ICI: Any medical procedure that has harms as well as benefits needs to be preceded by a *full informed consent procedure*.

When applied to the case of expansion of newborn screening, the fact that expansion of newborn screening will possibly lead to an increase in harms, will lead a defender of the ICI to conclude that this procedure has to be preceded by a full informed consent procedure. From now on, when I refer to the ICI, I will refer to this specific application in the case of expanded newborn screening program.

The proponent of the ICI will state that, as the screening offer expands and becomes more controversial, the informed consent procedure becomes more important. The main underlying normative assumption of this claim must be a notion of a right to an autonomous decision.

Of course, more pragmatic reasons for acquiring informed consent can be mentioned, such as an epistemological concern to determine what is best to do in a specific case. However, such considerations do not suffice as a defence of the ICI. The ICI is not in the first place defended because people would know best what is good for them, and that therefore they are best equipped to make a good decision. If this was the claim, then the possibility of other people deciding could still be left open, for example in cases where the individual lacked the required expertise. So the claim must be that such decisions should be left to people themselves, and not be forced upon them, *independent* from the question whether this is the 'best' choice.

Therefore, if the ICI is to be any more than a pragmatic decision procedure about what is best, it needs to hold that there is something morally objectionable about the pre-empting of people's choices. The ICI presumes that a good informed consent procedure is of intrinsic importance whenever there is the possibility of significant harms and benefits. Therefore, this view derives its plausibility from the claim that the only one who is authorized to make important (health) decisions in someone's life is the person concerned, or in the case of newborn screening, the parents.

[10] Note that although it is crucial here that newborn screening is a medical activity, this does not mean that all the harms (or the benefits for that matter) that play a role here need to be of a *medical* nature.

The claim is that whenever a medical procedure might turn out to be disadvantageous it is required that there be a *real* or *full* informed consent procedure, as opposed to an informed consent procedure that is mainly symbolic or procedural. To do otherwise is considered as an unjustified invasion in people's lives. It is therefore crucial to note that, according to the proponent of the ICI, to refrain from attaining informed consent is to infringe on the right to the freedom from unconsented invasive interventions by others.

So the proponent of the ICI will argue that we should give the parents sufficient information and then let parents decide in order to attain full informed consent. Let us see what this may entail. How do we achieve full informed consent?

12.3. Full Informed Consent

If newborn screening calls for full informed consent, how could this be achieved? What aspects of an informed consent procedure are important to prevent the government (or anybody else) from intervening in people's health choices?

In this section I will assume that the current informed consent procedures in different countries would be unsatisfactory to the proponent of the ICI, at least if the program were expanded. The informed consent procedure needs to be improved or strengthened.

It seems natural when we think of 'improving' an informed consent procedure, to think along two lines of improvement, information and consent. Improvement along the line of information could include the amount of information, the comprehensiveness of the information and the actual comprehension of the subjects. Improvement along the lines of consent may be that subjects have more options, are better aware of making a choice or feel less pressure in making a certain choice.[11]

12.3.1. Information

Assuming that the current informed consent procedure for newborn screening is insufficient, how could we improve it?

---

[11] See Faden and Beauchamp (1986), who analyze informed consent into the following components: disclosure, comprehension, voluntariness, competence, and consent.

Concerning the content of the information I see three possibilities. First, it may be suggested that the expansion of the screening program necessitates the provision of *more* information, simply by giving a more complete description of the diseases involved, data on the symptoms, the treatment options, the prevalence and so on. This should enable parents to get information as to what screening involves, and to consider what drawbacks might be involved. The immediate problem that arises, particularly if screening is performed on twenty or more diseases, is that this would soon lead to an information overload. So it might be that by giving more information, people would be less informed.

Secondly, there is the 'category approach', which is less drastic. This would entail that instead of trying to give specific information on specific diseases, the diseases could be categorized according to several criteria. So different types of diseases (e.g. serious/not so serious, treatable/not treatable, etc.) could then be described and this would make it easier for parents to decide what their preferences are. This would imply that one decides what features are relevant, and then proceeds to map diseases accordingly, so for example DMD would then fall under the category of serious, untreatable, monofactorial diseases, with an onset longer than two years. The question however is whether each of the diseases can be classified so easily. There is evidence, for example, that another candidate disease for screening, Cystic Fibrosis (CF), develops symptoms differently in different patients. There appears to be a continuum between very serious, and barely without symptoms (Kerr 2000). How should such a disease be classified?

The supposition in the category approach is that by presenting the information, the relevant considerations for choosing one way or the other will be clear. But this is not necessarily so. So a third alternative could be not only to describe different categories, but also to mention different types of considerations. So instead of mentioning that DMD is an untreatable, hereditary disease, that has an onset longer than two years, it could be mentioned that screening for DMD might have reproductive benefits (the prevention of a second child with this disease). The advantage would be that people do not miss arguments they might not have thought of themselves. The disadvantage could however be that by presenting the relevant considerations, we would clearly abandon the demand of non-directiveness, which is often seen as necessary component of autonomous choice. The relevance of the arguments would in this case be given in advance. Not every proponent of the ICI would be comfortable with this non-neutral approach.

Apart from the questions related to which approach to take and how much and what type of information is appropriate, there is a separate question concerning the actual comprehension. People have to understand to some extent what the procedure entails. We want them to understand, not just to take the information for granted. It has been mentioned that the first few days after giving birth to a child is not an ideal time for parents to process information—and to think about what this information may mean. So the informed consent procedure may benefit from informing parents at an earlier stage than that, for example, during pregnancy. That way parents would probably be more thoroughly aware of the choice they are making when consenting to screening. Since this is intended as a way to strengthen the informed consent procedure, it requires a significantly greater effort of the health professional in providing information. It does not suffice to just hand out brochures, or to use ways of informing parents that only reach a part of the population. If this is to be a part of the informed consent procedure all parents should encounter this information.

12.3.2. Consent/Choice

Now suppose that the measures suggested in the previous section are successful. We have better informed parents. Now what? If the point of departure is that information serves as a way to enable people to make better choices, we should now focus our attention on consent.

The informed consent procedure could be strengthened by focussing attention on the consent process through making people more aware of the fact that they are making a choice. Two ways to achieve this are by being very explicit about the possibility of refusal and by requiring the parents to mail the blood sample themselves (Parsons et al. 2000).

The next question is: consent to what? How much choice should parents have? This could take at least four forms. The first and most simple way is to emphasize the consent or dissent itself. In this approach there would be a 'take it or leave it' policy. Either people have their child screened for all diseases in the program, or for none at all. Although this suffices for a small and homogeneous program, it clearly will not do for a more diverse and large one. The fact that somebody wants his child screened for PKU in no way implies that he wants his child screened for DMD.

At the other extreme there is the possibility of parents choosing between a number of different diseases. Parents should then be able to choose what diseases they want their child to be screened for. Then parents could decide for themselves to have their child screened for PKU, but not DMD (or the other way around) and so on. Merely for practical reasons this seems an unattractive option too. When there are dozens of diseases offered it can not be expected that people will be able to make well-considered choice. Moreover, such a strategy would lead to an administrative disaster. For example, the mistakes made by laboratories are likely to increase significantly when everybody makes their own personal selection of diseases.

As I have already mentioned in the discussion of information, it would probably be more realistic to limit the choice between different categories. Then parents could choose between having their child screened for treatable conditions but not for untreatable conditions, or for carrier status but not for susceptibilities. This is the category approach to choice.

Even more simplified the choice could also be limited to a standard screening program and an additional optional category of controversial diseases. However such an approach would deviate from what the ICI seems to require, since the different controversial diseases are controversial for very different reasons. Therefore the same argument applies as in the 'take it or leave it' policy. When parents indicate that they want their child screened for DMD this does not imply that they want to know about susceptibilities for allergies as well.

12.3.3. Information and Choice

It is important to stress that the different ways of strengthening the informed consent procedure are not merely optional to the proponent of the ICI. Instead they follow from the ICI. A stronger focus on information *and* consent is not merely required because information may be interesting, or because giving explicit consent gives people a good feeling. The proponent of the ICI of course needs to say more. As I remarked before, in order to claim that there is an intrinsic connection between possible harms and the requirement of informed consent, the proponent of the ICI needs to hold that in the absence of such a procedure we do not only fear that harm will be done, but that such an intervention infringes the right of the subject to be free from such an intervention. From this it follows that merely supplying more information will not do, nor will merely giving more options. More information does not promote autonomy, unless the possibility of choice is added. And, conversely, choice cannot be autonomous, unless people are well informed. So, there is an *internal* connection in the ICI between the giving of information and the element of choice.

For this reason I have thus far spoken of full informed consent, instead of fully informed consent. I believe that the second formulation wrongly places an emphasis on merely supplying information, thereby supposing that consent will follow. I think this is in no way obvious. The proponent of the ICI will stress the importance of information *and* consent.

It is not necessary for the proponent of the ICI to hold that this information and choice need to be unlimited, in the sense that the people need to receive all the possible relevant information. A category approach will do. Since—for reasons stated above—I believe that this is the strongest version of the ICI, I will assume for the rest of this chapter that the proponent of the ICI will defend a version of the category approach.

12.4. Problems for the ICI

If it is true that the expansion of newborn screening necessitates full informed consent, we are faced with an immediate practical problem. It turns out that it is very difficult to get parents to take an active stance on these matters. Newborn screening is an issue that most people never think about before they are confronted with it, and often not even then. Parents generally do not take the time to understand what risks or drawbacks are involved (Hosli et al. forthcoming). This seems a problem for comprehension.

Related to this is the problem that it is very difficult, not to say impossible, not to directly influence people's choice when supplying this sort of information (Clarke 1991). The mere fact that a possibility to screen exists, presents itself to parents as a reason to assume that this screening is worthwhile. Since screening is performed on an entire population, and is conducted routinely, it is even more difficult not to influence the outcome of the deliberation of the parents, and to neutrally present the information. This is a problem for the ICI because the link between information and choice that I made, presupposes that people will be able to make up their own mind. If all we want is people to do what is suggested, we do not want full informed consent, but only that people do not complain.

The solution to these problems, so the proponent of the ICI will propose, is to become more active in counselling, in other words to make informed consent feasible by strengthening the informed consent procedure. But this is only possible at the expense of the non-intrusiveness of screening. When the informed consent procedure is organized so that these problems are surmounted, the screening procedure itself has become too burdensome. There are three reasons for this.

Firstly there is the *burden of information* itself. This burden becomes unacceptably high. Even if we embrace the category approach to information, there is still a vast amount of information to be processed. If we really want parents to be informed we need at least a description of what different types of diseases there are, what carrier status is, what treatment means in this context, and so on. This cannot be done in a few words, and requires an attentive study by each individual, which seems excessive, since only for one in a thousand or so will the outcome of the test be relevant.

There is even a stronger case to be made here. Even if there were only one category that people had to be informed about, the presumption of the ICI is that there are real advantages and disadvantages. A minimal requirement therefore is that these advantages and disadvantages become clear to the person who consents. It follows that information cannot stop at the point where it is claimed that there is a procedure and that it serves a purpose. The ICI requires a certain complexity of information. This, in combination with the notion of comprehension imposes a very large burden of information, and hence an active role for the professional in providing that information.

Connected to, but distinct from, the problem of the burden of information is the *burden of choice*. When the parents have processed the information, they are expected to make a choice. Presuming that the informed consent brochure doesn't supply an argumentation, they will have to sort out the relevant arguments, and find out for themselves which argument should prevail. And then they have to make a choice. This burden of choice becomes larger as the decision to be taken becomes more controversial. And the decision whether or not to screen *is* controversial for some diseases—uncommon as they may be.

A third problem for the ICI is *medicalization* (Verweij 2000: 69–95). When health care professionals actively seek consent or dissent, people will be pressed to make up their mind. Medicalization is a consequence of having to choose in this situation. Worries will arise that weren't there before. Whilst such screening is aimed at detecting serious diseases we are also dealing with extremely rare ones. So we may suppose that for most people, none of these diseases will be part of their perception of the world. This will be likely to change at least to an extent when they are pressed to think about the consequences of screening. A full informed consent procedure may cause unnecessary anxiety and impact negatively upon parental well-being. Therefore, an active informed consent procedure is—at least in some way—an intrusion in the daily life of otherwise healthy people and may cause a different—medicalized—perception of the world.

Now the proponent of the ICI could try to play out the trumping character of the right to autonomy and argue that although there are indeed disadvantages and practical difficulties, they are on a different level than the right to autonomy, which is in a sense absolute.

But here an immediate problem appears. The person that is being screened (the infant) is not the same as the person who gives the consent (generally the parents). So the claim that unconsented screening is an intervention in the private life of people raises the question *whose* private life: that of the child, or that of the parents? This forces a proponent of the ICI to make a choice. Either he has to say that the person screened is not the person whose interest is served—and potentially harmed—by screening. Or he has to say that this is a case of proxy consent. In either scenario autonomy loses its trumping character. In the first scenario the 'intervention' (the giving of information) with respect to the parents is clearly non-medical, and therefore (according to the ICI) different standards apply than in a clinical medical context. In the second scenario, that of proxy consent, the right to autonomy loses its absolute character, since it is not obvious that parents will decide what the child would decide, when competent. Furthermore, it seems a stretch to say that one child will benefit from the same information that will damage another child.

12.5. Concluding Remarks

I think that the doubts raised in the previous section sufficiently illustrate that the ICI, when applied to expanded newborn screening, is not an attractive position. The least demanding version of full informed consent—the category approach—still places too much burden on society in general and parents in particular. What does this mean for newborn screening? Should we loosen the requirements of informed consent, or does it mean that expansion itself becomes problematic?

Given that a policy where only a few diseases are being screened leads to few complaints from the population (or from ethicists, or anyone else for that matter) the last conclusion seems a tempting one. The impossibility and undesirability of full informed consent when a lot of different types of diseases are being screened could give us an argument to restrict screening for diseases that fit the criteria of Wilson and Jungner, that is, diseases that are minimally controversial. It may appear that informed consent would then be unproblematic and so my objections would be met. The ICI would then stay intact, but it would force us to be more modest in our screening ambitions.

However, I believe that this conclusion is too easily reached. Although there is something to be said for a limited offer, I think it is important to note that in this case the parents' choice is being pre-empted too, which was exactly what the ICI was set up to prevent. If we choose not to screen for DMD, this means that we have decided not to attain information on the health of a child, which could have been attained very easily and cheaply. Given that our premise was that screening for DMD is controversial, this means that a choice has been made not to know where some people would have preferred to know. In other words, there is no way of offering screening that is neutral to the preferences of parents. This means that, although the option not to expand the screening program may be an attractive one, it does not offer an escape route for the proponent of the ICI.

This leads to the conclusion of this essay, which is that since for newborn screening full informed consent is neither feasible, nor desirable, we have to let go of the ICI. Whenever screening is offered, lives are being interfered with. The challenge is to find the best way to do so. The ICI may delude us into thinking that the difficulties of the policy maker to decide what diseases should be screened for, can be resolved by leaving the choice to individual parents. This, however, would be to walk away from the responsibility that a policy maker has.

This is not an argument *against* informed consent in newborn screening programs. What it does suggest is that not every choice in the medical field can be left up to the individual. The ICI fails to acknowledge that some medical interventions, such as (universal) newborn screening, are of an essentially collective character. Individual choice is not a panacea against the problems that arise when such a program does not exclusively bring blessings. This leads to the conclusion that we will probably end up with a screening program that not everybody *would* agree with. But this is still preferable to a program that places disproportional burdens on society, and that therefore nobody *could* reasonably agree to.

REFERENCES

Acheson, D. (1988). *Public Health in England*, Cmnd 289. London: HMSO.

Acheson, D. (1998). *Independent Inquiry into Inequalities in Health*. London: Stationery Office.

Ackerman, F. and Heinzerling, L. (2004). *Priceless: On Knowing the Price of Everything and the Value of Nothing*. New York: The New Press.

Adler, N. E. and Newman, K. (2002). 'Socioeconomic Disparities in Health: Pathways and Policies'. *Health Affairs*, 21: 60−76.

Allen, A. L. and Regan, M. C. Jr. (eds.) (1998). *Debating Democracy's Discontent*. Oxford: Oxford University Press.

American Academy of Pediatrics. (2002). *Guidelines for Perinatal Care* (5th edn). Elk Grove Village, IL: AAP.

American College of Obstetricians and Gynecologists and American College of Medical Genetics. (2001). *Preconception and Prenatal Carrier Screening for Cystic Fibrosis: Clinical and Laboratory Guidelines*. Washington, DC: ACOG/ACMG.

Anand, S., Peter, F., and Sen, A. (eds.) (2004). *Public Health, Ethics, and Equity*. Oxford: Oxford University Press.

Anderson, B. (1991). *Imagined Communities: Reflections on the Origin and Spread of Nationalism*. New York: Verso.

Annas, G. (2002). 'Bioterrorism, Public Health, and Civil Liberties'. *New England Journal of Medicine*, 346: 1337−42.

Arendt, H. (1973). *On Revolution*. New York: Viking.

Arneson, R. (1982). 'The Principle of Fairness and Free-rider Problems'. *Ethics*, 92(4): 616−33.

Asada, Y. and Hedemann, T. (2002). 'A Problem with the Individual Approach in the WHO Health Inequality Measurement'. *International Journal for Equity in Health*, 1(2).

Asch, P. and Gigliotti, A. (1991). 'The Free-Rider Paradox: Theory, Evidence, and Teaching'. *Journal of Economic Education*, Winter: 33−8.

Ashcraft, R. (1986). *Revolutionary Politics and Locke's Two Treatises of Government*. Princeton: Princeton University Press.

Ashton, J. and Seymour. H. (1988). *The New Public Health*. Milton Keynes: Open University Press.

Atkinson, A. B. (1970). 'On the Measurement of Inequality'. *Journal of Economic Theory*, 2: 244−63.

Austoker, J. (1999). 'Gaining Informed Consent for Screening'. *British Medical Journal*, 319: 722–3.

Bailyn, B. (1965). *The Ideological Origins of the American Revolution*. Cambridge, MA: Harvard University Press.

Bale, J. F. (2002). 'Congenital Infections'. *Neurologic Clinics*, 20(4): 1039–60.

Barber, B. (1974). *The Death of Communal Liberty*. Princeton, NJ: Princeton University Press.

Barendregt, J., Bonneux, L., and van der Maas, P. (1997). 'The Health Care Costs of Smoking'. *New England Journal of Medicine*, 337:1052–7.

Baron, H. (1966). *The Crisis of the Early Italian Renaissance* (2nd ed.). Princeton: Princeton University Press.

Baron, S., Field, J., and Schuller, T. (eds.) (2000). *Social Capital: Critical Perspectives*. Oxford: Oxford University Press.

Barry, B. (1965). *Political Argument*. London: Routlege & Kegan Paul.

Barry, B. (2005). *Why Social Justice Matters*. Cambridge: Polity Press.

Bates, B. (2003). 'Prenatal Screening Halves CF births: Data from Large Screening Program'. *OB/Gyn News*, (15 December 2003). Available at: http://www.findarticles.com/p/articles/mi_m0CYD/is_24_38/ai_112404383 (accessed 7/2/06).

Bayer, R. (1991). *Private Acts, Social Consequences: AIDS and the Politics of Public Health*. New Brunswick, NJ: Rutgers University Press.

Bayer, R. and Healton, C. (1989). 'Controlling AIDS in Cuba. The Logic of Quarantine'. *New England Journal of Medicine*, 320/15: 1022–4.

Bayer, R., Gostin, L.O., and Magraw, D. (1995). 'Trades, AIDS, and the Public's Health: the Limits of Economic Analysis'. *Georgetown Law Journal*, 83: 79–107.

Beaglehole, R. (ed.) (2003). *Global Public Health: A New Era*. Oxford: Oxford University Press.

Beauchamp, D. (1976). 'Public Health as Social Justice'. *Inquiry*, 12: 3–14.

Beauchamp, D. (1985). 'Community: The Neglected Tradition of Public Health'. *Hastings Center Report*; 15(6): 28–36.

Beauchamp, D. and Steinbock, B. (eds.) (1999). *New Ethics for the Public's Health*. Oxford: Oxford University Press.

Beauchamp, D. E. (1988). *The Health of the Republic: Epidemics, Medicine, and Moralism as Challenges to Democracy*. Philadelphia, PA: Temple University Press.

Beauchamp, T. and Childress, J. (1979). *Principles of Biomedical Ethics* (1st ed.). Oxford: Oxford University Press.

Beauchamp, T. and Childress, J. (2001). *Principles of Biomedical Ethics* (5th ed.). Oxford: Oxford University Press.

Bennett, R. and Erin, C. A. (eds.) (1999). *HIV and AIDS: Testing, Screening, and Confidentiality*. Oxford: Oxford University Press.

Bentham, J. (1996). In H.L.A. Hart and and F. Rosen (eds.) *Introduction to the Principles of Morals and Legislation.* Oxford: Clarendon Press.

Berlin, I. ([1958] 1969). 'Two Concepts of Liberty'. In *Four Essays on Liberty.* New York: Oxford, pp. 118–72.

Bidmeade, I. and Reynolds, C. (1997). *Public Health Law in Australia: its Current State and Future Directions.* Canberra: Commonwealth of Australia.

Braveman, P., Starfield, B., and Geiger, H. J. (2001). 'World Health Report 2000: How it Removes Equity from the Agenda for Public Health Monitoring and Policy'. *British Medical Journal,* 323: 678–81.

Brock, D. W. (1989). 'Justice, Health Care, and the Elderly'. *Philosophy & Public Affairs,* 18(3): 297–312.

Brock, D. W. (1995). 'Justice and the ADA: Does Prioritizing and Rationing Health Care Discriminate Against the Disabled?'. *Social Philosophy and Policy,* 12: 159–84.

Brock, D. W. (2000). 'Health Care Resource Prioritization and Discrimination Against Persons with Disabilities', in L. Francis and A. Silvers (eds.) *Americans with Disabilities: Implications for Individuals and Institutions.* New York: Routledge.

Brock, D. W. (2002). 'Priority to the Worst Off in Health Care Resource Prioritization,' in M. Battin, R. Rhodes, and A. Silvers (eds.) *Medicine and Social Justice.* New York: Oxford University Press

Brock, D. W. (2003a). 'Ethical Issues in the Use of Cost Effectiveness Analysis for the Prioritization of Health Care Resources', in T. Tan-Torres Edejer, R. Baltussen, T. Adam et al. (eds.) *Making Choices in Health: WHO Guide to Cost-Effectiveness Analysis.* Geneva: World Health Organization.

Brock, D. W. (2003b). 'Separate Spheres and Indirect Benefits'. *Cost-Effectiveness and Resource Allocation,* 1: 4.

Brock, D. W. (2004a). 'Ethical Issues in the Use of Cost Effectiveness Analysis for the Prioritization of Health Care Resources', in G. Khusfh (ed.) *Handbook of Bioethics: Taking Stock of the Field from a Philosophical Perspective.* Dordrecht: Kluwer Publishers.

Brock, D. W. (2004b). 'Ethical Issues in the Use of Cost Effectiveness Analysis for the Prioritization of Health Care Resources', in S. Anand, A. Peter, and A. Sen (eds.) *Public Health, Ethics and Equity.* Oxford: Oxford University Press.

Brock, D. W. and Daniels, N. (1994) 'Ethical Foundations of the Clinton Administration's Proposed Health Care System'. *Journal of American Medical Association,* 271: 1189–96.

Brock, D. and Wikler, D. (2006). 'Ethical Issues in Resource Allocation, Research, and New Product Development', in D. T. Jamison and J. G. Breman (eds.) *Disease Control Priorities in Developing Countries* (2nd edn). Oxford: Oxford University Press.

Buchanan, D. (2000). *An Ethic for Health Promotion: Rethinking the Sources of Human Well-Being.* Oxford: Oxford University Press.

Buchanan, A., Brock, D., Daniels, N., and Wikler, D. (2000) *From Chance to Choice: Genes and Justice*. Cambridge: Cambridge University Press.

Burris, S. (1997). 'The Invisibility of Public Health: Population-Level Measures in a Politics of Market Individualism'. *American Journal of Public Health*, 87: 1607–10.

Callahan, D. and Jennings, B. (2002). 'Ethics and Public Health: Forging a Strong Relationship'. *American Journal of Public Health*, 92(2): 169–76.

Campbell, E., and Ross, L. F. (2005). 'Parental Attitudes and Beliefs Regarding the Genetic Testing of Children'. *Community Genetics*, 8(2): 94–102.

Capron, A.M. and Reis, A. (2005). 'Designing an Equitable Strategy for Allocating Antiretroviral Treatments'. *PLoS Medicine*. 2(3): 69.

Carman, W. F., Elder, A. G., Wallace, L. A. et al. (2000). 'Effects of Influenza Vaccination of Health Care Workers on Mortality of Elderly People in Long-term Care: A Randomized Controlled Trial'. *Lancet*, 355(9198): 93–7.

Casey, C., Vellozzi, C., Mootrey, G. T. et al. (Vaccinia Case Definition Development Working Group, Advisory Committee on Immunization Practices-Armed Forces Epidemiological Board Smallpox Vaccine Safety Working Group) (2006). 'Surveillance Guidelines for Smallpox Vaccine (Vaccinia) Adverse Reactions'. *Morbidity and Mortality Weekly Report*, 55: 1–16.

CDC (Centers for Disease Control and Prevention) (2002a). *Public Health's Infrastructure: a Status Report*. Atlanta: CDC.

CDC (Centers for Disease Control and Prevention) (2002b). 'Congenital Syphilis—United States 2002'. *Morbidity and Mortality Weekly Report*, 53: 716–19.

CDC (Centers for Disease Control and Prevention) (2002c). 'STDs in Women and Infants, 2002', *National STD Surveillance Report*. Atlanta, GA: CDC. Available at: http://www.cdc.gov/std/stats02/women&inf.htm (accessed 15/3/06).

CDC (Centers for Disease Control and Prevention) (2003). 'Sexually transmitted disease Surveillance Supplement'. *Syphilis Surveillance Report 2002*. Atlanta, GA: CDC. Available from: www.cdc.gov/std/stats02/syphilis.htm (accessed 7/2/06).

CESCR (Committee on Economic, Social and Cultural Rights) (2000). 'The Right to the Highest Attainable Standard of Health'. General Comment 14, E/C.12/2000/4, 4 July. Available at: www.unhchr.ch/tbs/doc.nsf/(accessed 23/3/06).

Chadwick, E. (1965) *Report on the Sanitary Condition of the Labouring Population of Great Britain*. Edinburgh: University Press.

Childress, J. F., Faden, R. R., Gaare, R. D. et al. (2002). 'Public Health: Mapping the Terrain'. *Journal of Law, Medicine & Ethics*, 30: 170–8.

Clarke, A. (1991). 'Is Non-directive Counselling Possible?' *Lancet*, 335: 1145–7.

Coles, F. B., Balzano, G. J., and Morse, D. J. (1992). 'An Outbreak of Influenza A (H3N2) in a Well Immunized Nursing Home Population'. *Journal of the American Geriatrics Society*, 40: 589–92.

Commission on Macroeconomics and Health (2001). *Macroeconomics and Health: Investing in Health for Economic Development*. Geneva: World Health Organization.

Cribb, A. (2005). *Health and the Good Society: Setting Healthcare Ethics in Social Context*. Oxford: Oxford University Press.

Cullity, G. (1995). 'Moral Free Riding'. *Philosophy and Public Affairs*, 24(1): 3–34.

Daniels, N. (1985). *Just Health Care*. Cambridge: Cambridge University Press.

Daniels, N. (1988). *Am I My Parents' Keeper? An Essay on Justice Between the Young and the Old*. New York: Oxford University Press.

Daniels, N. (1998). 'Distributive Justice and the Use of Summary Measures of Population Health Status', in Institute of Medicine (ed.) *Summarizing Population Health: Directions for the Development and Application of Population Metrics*. Washington DC: Institute of Medicine.

Daniels, N. (2004). 'How to Achieve Fair Distribution of ARTs in '3 by 5': Fair Process and Legitimacy in Patient Selection'. Paper prepared for Consultation on Equitable Access to Care for HIV/AIDS, World Health Organization, Geneva. 26–7 January.

Daniels, N. (2005). 'Fair Process in Patient Selection for Antiretroviral Treatment in WHO's Goal of 3 by 5'. *Lancet*, 366: 169–71.

Daniels, N., Light, D., and Caplan, R. L. (1996). *Benchmarks of Fairness for Health Care Reform*. Oxford: Oxford University Press.

Daniels, N., Kennedy, B. P., and Kawachi, I. (1999). 'Why Justice is Good for Our Health: the Social Determinants of Health Inequalities'. *Daedalus*, 128(Fall): 215–51.

Daniels, N., Kennedy, B., and Kawachi, I. (2000a). 'Justice is Good for Our Health'. *Boston Review*, 25(1): 6–15.

Daniels, N., Kawachi, I. and Kennedy, B. (2000b). *Is Inequality Bad For Our Health?* Boston, MA: Beacon Press.

Dare, T. (1998). 'Mass Immunisations Programmes: Some Philosophical Issues'. *Bioethics*, 12(2): 125–49.

Dawson, A. (2005). 'The Determination of "Best Interests" in Relation to Childhood Vaccinations'. *Bioethics*, 19(2): 187–205.

Dawson, A. (forthcoming). 'What are the Moral Obligations of the Traveller in Relation to Vaccination?' *Journal of Travel Medicine & Infectious Disease*.

Deaton, A. (2002). 'Policy Implications of the Gradient of Health and Wealth'. *Health Affairs*, 21: 13–30.

De Cock, D. M., Mbori-Ngacha, D., and Marum. E. (2002). 'Shadow on the Continent: Public Health and HIV/AIDS in Africa in the 21st Century'. *Lancet*, 360: 67–72.

Department of Health and Human Services. (2000). *Healthy People 2010*. Washington, DC: Government Printing Office.

Diggins, J. P. (1984). *The Lost Soul of American Politics: Virtue, Self-interest, and the Foundation of Liberalism*. New York: Basic Books.

Donaldson, C. (1999). 'Valuing the Benefits of Publicly-Provided Health Care: Does "Ability to Pay" Preclude the use of "Willingness to Pay"?'. *Social Science and Medicine*, 49(4): 551–63.

Downie, R. S., Fyfe, C., and Tannahill, A. (1990). *Health Promotion: Models and Values*. Oxford: Oxford University Press.

Draper, H. and Sorell, T. (2002). 'Patients' Responsibilities in Medical Ethics.' *Bioethics*, 16: 335–52.

Duffy, J. (1990). *The Sanitarians: a History of American Public Health*. Urbana and Chicago: University of Illinois Press.

Epstein, R. A. (2003). 'Let the Shoemaker Stick to his Last: a Defense of the "Old" Public Health'. *Perspectives in Biology and Medicine*, 46(S3): S138–59.

Erbe, R. W. and Levy, H. L. (1996). 'Neonatal Screening', in D. L. Rimoin, J. M. Connor, and R. E. Pyeritz (eds.) *Emery and Rimoin's Principles and Practice of Medical Genetics* (3rd edn). London: Churchill Livingston, pp. 581–93.

Ewing, R., Schimd, T., Killingsworth, R., Zlot, A., and Raudenbush, S. (2003) 'Relationship Between Urban Sprawl and Physical Activity, Obesity, and Morbidity'. *American Journal of Health Promotion*, 18(1): 47–57.

Faden, R. R. and Beauchamp, T. L. (1986). *A History and Theory of Informed Consent*. Oxford: Oxford University Press.

Feinberg, J. (1973). *Social Philosophy*. Englewood Cliffs, NJ: Prentice Hall.

Feinberg, J. (1984). *Harm to Others*. Oxford: Oxford University Press.

Feinberg, J. (1986). *Harm to Self*. Oxford: Oxford University Press.

Fidler, D. P. (1999). *International Law and Infectious Diseases*. Oxford: Clarendon Press.

Forester, J. (1989). *Planning in the Face of Power*. Berkeley: University of California Press.

Forester, J. (1999). *The Deliberative Practitioner: Encouraging Participatory Planning Processes*. Cambridge, MA: MIT Press.

Fox, D. M. and Schaffer, D. C. (1991) 'Tax Administration as Health Policy'. *Journal of Health Politics and Policy Law*, 16: 251–60.

Frankena, W. (1973). *Ethics* (2nd ed). Engelwood Cliffs, NJ: Prentice-Hall.

Freeman, M. (ed.) (forthcoming). *The Ethics of Public Health: International Library of Medicine, Ethics and Law*. Ashgate.

Frenk, J. (1992). 'The New Public Health', in Pan American Health Organization (ed.) *The Crisis of Public Health: Reflections for Debate*. Washington, DC: PAHO/WHO.

Fried, C. (1970). *An Anatomy of Values: Problem of Personal and Social Choice*. Harvard: Harvard University Press.

Friedmann, J. (1987). *Planning in the Public Domain*. Princeton, NJ: Princeton University Press.

Gakidou, E. and King, G. (2002). 'Measuring Total Health Inequality: Adding Individual Variation to Group-Level Differences'. *International Journal for Equity in Health*, 1(3).

Garber, A. (1989). 'Pursuing the Links Between Socioeconomic Factors and Health', in D. S. Gomby and B.H. Kehrer (eds.) *Pathways to Health: the Role of Social Factors*. Menlo Park, CA: Kaiser Family Foundation.

Garland, M. (1992). 'Justice, Politics and Community: Expanding Access and Rationing Health Services in Oregon'. *Law, Medicine and Health Care*, 20: 70.

Garrard, E., and Dawson, A. (2005). 'What is the Role of the REC? Paternalism, Inducements and Harm in Research Ethics'. *Journal of Medical Ethics*, 31: 419–23.

Garrett, L. (2001). *Betrayal of Trust: The Collapse of Global Public Health*. Oxford: Oxford University Press.

General Accounting Office. (2003). *Newborn Screening: Characteristics of State Programs*. Report Number GAO-03–449. Washington, DC: GAO.

Gezondheidsraad (Dutch Health Council) (2005). *Neonatale Screening*. Den Haag: GR.

Gold, M., Siegel, J., Russell, L., and Weinstein, M. (eds.) (1996). *Cost-Effectiveness in Health and Medicine*. New York: Oxford University Press.

Goodin, R. (1989). *No Smoking: The Ethical Issues*. Chicago: University of Chicago Press.

Gostin, L. O. (2000a). 'Public Health Law in a New Century: Parts I–III'. *Journal of American Medical Association*, 283: 2837–41, 2979–84, 3118–22.

Gostin, L. O. (2000b). *Public Health Law: Power, Duty, Restraint*. Berkeley/New York: University of California Press/Milbank Memorial Fund.

Gostin, L. O. (2001). 'Public Health, Ethics, and Human Rights: A Tribute to the Late Jonathan Mann'. *Journal of Law, Medicine & Ethics*, 29:121–30.

Gostin, L. O. (2002a). *Public Health Law and Ethics: A Reader*. Berkeley, CA: University of California Press.

Gostin, L. O. (2002b). 'Public Health Law, Ethics, and Human Rights', in L.O. Gostin (ed.) *Public Health Law and Ethics: A Reader*. Berkeley, CA/New York, NY: University of California Press/The Milbank Memorial Fund.

Gostin, L. O. (2004a). 'Law and Ethics in Population Health', *Australian & New Zealand Journal of Public Health*, 28: 7–12.

Gostin, L. O. (2004b). *The AIDS Pandemic: Complacency, Injustice, and Unfulfilled Expectations*. Chapel Hill: University of North Carolina Press.

Gostin, L. O. and Lazzarini, Z. (1997). *Human Rights and Public Health in the AIDS Pandemic*. New York: Oxford University Press.

Gostin L.O. and Bloche M. G. (2003). 'The Politics of Public Health: A Reply to Richard Epstein'. *Perspectives in Biology and Medicine*, 46(S3): S160–S175.

Green, M. D. and Botkin, J. R. (2003). ' "Genetic Exceptionalism" in Medicine: Clarifying the Differences between Genetic and Nongenetic Tests'. *Annals of Internal Medicine*, 138: 571–5.

Green, D. P. and Shapiro, I. (1994). *Pathologies of Rational Choice Theory*. New Haven: Yale University Press.

Griffiths, S. and Hunter, D. (1999). 'Introduction', in S. Griffiths and D. Hunter (eds.) *Perspectives in Public Health*. Oxford: Radical Medical Press.

Halévy, E. (1966). *The Growth of Philosophical Radicalism*. Boston: Beacon.

Hamlin, C. (2002). 'The History and Development of Public Health in Developed Countries', in R. Detels, J. McEwen, R. Beaglehole, and H. Tanaka (eds.) *Oxford Textbook of Public Health* (4th ed). Oxford: Oxford University Press.

Hardin, G. (1968). 'The Tragedy of the Commons'. *Science*, 13 December 13, 162: 1243–8.

Harlan, Justice John (1905). US Supreme Court Decision: *Jacobson v. Massachusetts* 25 S. Ct. 358.

Harré, R. (1998). *The Singular Self*. London: Sage Publications.

Hart, H. L. A. (1955). 'Are There any Natural Rights?' *The Philosophical Review*, 64(2): 175–91.

Hartz, L. (1955). *The Liberal Tradition in America: An Interpretation of American Political Thought since the Revolution*. New York: Harcourt, Brace.

Health Council of the Netherlands (2003). *The Impact of Passive Smoking on Public Health*. The Hague: Health Council of the Netherlands.

Heijnen, M-L., Waldboer, Q., Siedenburg, E. et al. (2004). 'Hepatitis-B-vaccinatiecampagne gedragsgebonden risicogroepen op koers' (HBV vaccination campaign for behavioural risk groups on schedule). *Infectieziekten Bulletin*, 15: 342–8.

Heinzerling, L. (1998). 'Regulatory Costs of Mythic Proportions'. *Yale Law Journal*, 107: 1981–2070.

Hermerén, G. (1999). 'Neonatal Screening: Ethical Aspects'. *Acta Paediatrica Supplement*, 432: 99–103.

Holland, W. W. and Stewart, S. (1997). *Public Health: the Vision and the Challenge*. London: Nuffield Trust.

Hollier, L. M., Hill, J., Sheffield, J. S., and Wendel, G. D. (2003). 'State Laws Regarding Prenatal Syphilis Screening in the United States'. *American Journal of Obstetrics and Gynecology*. 184: 1178–83.

Hosli, E., Detmar, S., Dijkstra, N., Nijsingh, N., and Verweij, M. (forthcoming). 'Parental Preferences Towards Expanding the Neonatal Screening Programme'. Leiden: TNO Quality of Life.

Horsman, J., Furlong, W., Feeney, D., and Torrance, G. (2003). 'The Health Utilities Index (HUI): Concepts, Measurement Properties and Applications'. *Health Quality Life Outcomes*, 1(1): 54.

Institute of Medicine (1988). *The Future of Public Health*. Washington, DC: National Academy Press.

Institute of Medicine (1999). *Vaccines for the 21st Century: A Tool for Decision Making*. Washington, DC: National Academies Press.

Institute of Medicine (2001). *Health and Behavior:The Interplay of Biological, Behavioral, and Societal Influences*. Washington, DC: National Academy Press.

Institute of Medicine (2003). *The Future of the Public's Health in the Twenty First Century*. Washington, DC: National Academy Press.

Institute of Medicine (2004). *Immunization Safety Review: Vaccines And Autism*. Washington, DC: National Academic Press.

Jackson, R. J. (2003). 'The Impact of the Built Environment on Health: an Emerging Field'. *American Journal of Public Health*, 93: 1382−3.

Jacoby, R. (1987). *The Last Intellectuals*. New York: Farrar, Straus, and Giroux.

Jennings, B. (1981). 'Tradition and the Politics of Remembering'. *The Georgia Review*, XXXVI(1): 167−82.

Jennings, B. (2003a). 'On Authority and Justification in Public Health'. *Florida Law Review*, 55: 1241−56.

Jennings, B. (2003b). 'Frameworks for Ethics in Public Health'. *Acta Bioethica*, 9(2): 165−76.

Kagan, S. (1989). *The Limits of Morality*. Oxford: Clarendon Press.

Kant, I. ([1788] 1956). *Critique of Pure Reaso*, L.W. Beck (trans.) New York: Macmillan.

Kant, I. (1797). *The Metaphysics of Morals*. In M. J. Gregor (ed.) *Practical Philosophy: The Cambridge Edition of the Works of Immanuel Kant*. Cambridge: Cambridge University Press.

Kass, N. E. (2001). 'An Ethics Framework for Public Health'. *American Journal of Public Health*, 91(11): 1776−82.

Kekes, J. (1997). 'A Question for Egalitarians'. *Ethics*, 107: 658−69.

Kellman, B. (2001). 'Biological Terrorism: Legal Measures for Preventing a Catastrophe'. *Harvard Journal of Law & Public Policy*, 24: 417−85.

Keohane, N. O. (1980). *Philosophy and the State in France*. Princeton, NJ: Princeton University Press.

Kerr, A. (2000). 'Constructing Genetic Disease: the Clinical Continuum between Cystic Fibrosis and Male Infertility'. *Social Studies of Science*, 30(6): 847−94.

Kerruish, N. J., and Robertson, S. P. (2005). 'Newborn Screening: New Developments, New Dilemmas'. *Journal of Medical Ethics*, 31: 393−8.

Kessel, A. (2006). *Air, the Environment and Public Health*. Cambridge: Cambridge University Press.

Kitagawa, E. M. and Hauser, P. M. (1973). *Differential Mortality in the United States: A Study of Socio-economic Epidemiology*. Cambridge, MA: Harvard University Press.

Klein, R. (1997). 'Defining a Package of Healthcare Services the NHS is Responsible for: The Case Against'. *British Medical Journal*, 314: 503−5.

Klosko, G. (1987). 'Presumptive Benefit, Fairness and Political Obligation'. *Philosophy and Public Affairs*, 16(3): 241−59.

Kohn, L. T., Corrigan, J. M., and Donaldson, M. S. (eds.) (2000). *To Err is Human: Building a Safer Health System*. Washington, DC: National Academy Press.

Korn, D. A. and Shaffner, H. J. (1999). 'Gambling and the Health of the Public: Adopting a Public Health Perspective'. *Journal of Gambling Studies*, 15: 289–365.

Kotalik, J. (2005). 'Preparing for an Influenza Pandemic: Ethical issues'. *Bioethics*. 19: 422–31.

Kramnick, I. (1990). *Republicanism and Bourgeois Radicalism*. Ithaca, NY: Cornell University Press.

Kumar, R. (2001). *Consensualism in Principle*. London: Routledge.

Lalonde, M. (1974). *A New Perspective on the Health of Canadians*. Ottawa: National Ministry of Health & Welfare.

Lantz, P. M., House, J. S., Lepkowski, J. M. et al. (1998). 'Socioeconomic Factors, Health Behaviors, and Mortality Results From a Nationally Representative Prospective Study of US Adults'. *Journal of American Medical Association*. 279: 1703–8.

Lautze, S., Leaning, J., Raven-Roberts, A., Kent, R., and Mazurana, D. (2004). 'Assistance, Protection, and Governance Networks in Complex Emergencies'. *Lancet*, 364: 2134–41.

Lazaro, A. (2002). 'Theoretical Arguments for the Discounting of Health Consequences: Where Do We Go from Here?'. *Pharmacoeconomics*, 20: 943–61.

Lecluyese, A. and Cleemput, I. (2005). 'Making Health Continuous: Implications of Different Methods on the Measurement of Inequality'. *Health Economics*, 15: 99–104;

Leichter, H. (2003). ' "Evil Habits" and "Personal Choices": Assigning Responsibility for Health in the 20th Century'. *Milbank Quarterly*, 81(4): 603–26.

Levy, J. I., Chemerynski, S. M., and Tuchmann, J. L. (2006). 'Incorporating Concepts of Inequality and Inequity into Health Benefits Analysis'. *International Journal for Equity in Health*, 28 March, 5(2).

Lipscomb, J., Weinstein, M., and Torrance, G. (1996). 'Time Preference,' in M. Gold, J. Siegel, L. Russell, and M. Weinstein (eds.), *Cost-Effectiveness in Health and Medicine*. New York: Oxford University Press.

Littlewood, J. (2002). *The History of the Development of Cystic Fibrosis Care*. London: The UK CF Trust. Available at: http://www.cysticfibrosismedicine.com/public/articles_text.asp?id=108 (accessed 7/2/06).

Loeber, G., Webster, D., and Aznarez, A. (1999). 'Quality Evaluation of Newborn Screening Programs'. *Acta Paediatrica*, 432: 3–6.

Low, A. and Low, A. (2006). 'Importance of Relative Measures in Policy on Health Inequalities'. *British Medical Journal*, 332: 967–9.

Lynch, J., Smith, G. D., Harper, S. et al. (2004). 'Is Income Inequality a Determinant of Population Health? Part 1. A Systematic Review'. *Milbank Quarterly*, 82: 5–99.

Lynch, J. W., Kaplan, G. A., Pamuk, E. R. et al. (1998). 'Income Inequality and Mortality in Metropolitan Areas of the United States'. *American Journal of Public Health*, 88: 1074–9.

Mackenbach, J. (2004). 'The Development of a Strategy for Tackling Health Inequalities in the Netherlands'. *International Journal for Equity in Health*, 3: 11.

MacIntyre, A. (1981). *After Virtue*. South Bend, IN: University of Notre Dame Press.

Macklin, R. (2004). *Ethics and Equity in Access to HIV Treatment—3 by 5 Initiative*. Geneva: WHO. Available at: http://www.who.int/ethics/en/background-macklin.pdf (accessed 5/5/06).

Mann, J. M. (1997). 'Medicine and Public Health, Ethics and Human Rights'. *The Hastings Center Report*, (May—June) 27: 6—13.

Mann, J. M., Gruskin, S., Grodin, M. A., and Annas, G. J. (eds.) (1999). *Health and Human Rights: A Reader*. New York: Routledge.

Marchand, S. and Wikler, D. (2002). 'Health Inequalities and Justice', in J. Tao and L. Po-wah (eds.) *Cross-Cultural Perspectives on the (Im)possibility of Global Bioethics*. Dordrecht: Kluwer Academic Publishers, pp. 209—21.

Marchand, S., Wikler, D., and Landesman, B. (1998). 'Class, Health and Justice'. *Milbank Quarterly*, 76(3): 449—67.

Marmot, M. (2004). *The Status Syndrome*. New York: Henry Holt.

Marmot, M. G., Smith, G. D., and Stansfeld, S. (1991). 'Health Inequalities among British Civil Servants: the Whitehall II Study'. *Lancet*, 337(8754): 1387—93.

Marone, J. A. (1997). 'Enemies of the People: the Moral Dimension to Public Health'. *Journal of Health Politics, Policy and Law*, 22: 993—1020.

Marseille, E., Hofmann, P. B., and Kahn, J. G. (2002). 'HIV Prevention before HAART in Sub-Saharan Africa'. *Lancet*, 359: 1851—6.

Masaki, E., Green, R., Greig, F., Walsh, J., and Potts, M. (n.d.) 'Cost-effectiveness of HIV Interventions for Resource Scarce Countries: Setting Priorities for HIV/AIDS'. Available at: http://big.berkeley.edu/research.workingpapers.HIV_prev.revision1.03.pdf (accessed: 5/5/06).

Mathers, C. D., Murray, C. J. L., Salomon, J. A. et al. (2003). 'Healthy Life Expectancy: Comparison of OECD Countries in 2001'. *Australian and New Zealand Journal of Public Health*, 27: 5—11.

McMahan, J. (2002). *The Ethics of Killing*. New York: Oxford University Press.

Mellor, J. M. and Milyo, J. D. (2002). 'Income Inequality and Health Status in the United States'. *Journal of Human Resources*, 37: 510—39.

Menzel, P. (1990). *Strong Medicine: The Ethical Rationing of Health Care*. New York: Oxford University Press.

Menzel, P., Dolan, P., Richardson, J., and Olsen, J.A. (2002). 'The Role of Adaptation to Disability and Disease in Health State Valuation: A Preliminary Normative Analysis'. *Social Science and Medicine*, 55: 2149—58.

Mill, J. S. ([1859] 1974). *On Liberty*. Harmondsworth: Penguin.

Mills, C. W. (1959). *The Sociological Imagination*. New York: Oxford University Press.

Mohamed, K., Appleton, R., and Nicolaides, P. (2000). 'Delayed Diagnosis of Duchenne Muscular Dystrophy'. *European Journal of Paediatric Neurology*, 219–23.

Monaghan, S., Huws, D., and Navarro, M. (2003) *The Case for a New UK Health of the People Act*. London: The Nuffield Trust.

Morabia, A. and Zhang, F. F. (2004). 'History of Medical Screening: from Concepts to Action', *Postgraduate Medical Journal*, 80: 463–9.

Murphy, L. B. (2000). *Moral Demands in Nonideal Theory*. Oxford: Oxford University Press.

Murray, C. (1994). 'Quantifying the Burden of Disease: the Technical Basis for Disability Adjusted Life Years', in C. Murray and A. Lopez (eds.) *Global Comparative Assessments in the Health Sector: Disease Burden, Expenditures and Intervention Packages*. Geneva: World Health Organization.

Murray, C. (1996). 'Rethinking DALYs', in C. Murray and A Lopez (eds.). *The Global Burden of Disease: A Comprehensive Assessment of Morality and Disability from Diseases, Injuries, and Risk Factors in 1990 and Projected to 2020*. The Global Burden of Disease and Injury, Vol. 1. Cambridge MA: The Harvard School of Public Health.

Murray, C. J. L., Michaud, C. M., McKenna, M. T., and Marks, J. S. (1998). *U.S. Patterns of Mortality by County and Race: 1965–1994*. Cambridge, MA: Harvard Center for Population and Development Studies, 1–97.

Murray, C. J. L., Gakidou, E. E., and Frenk, J. (1999). 'Health Inequalities and Social Group Differences: What Should we Measure?' *Bulletin of the World Health Organization*, 77(7): 537–43.

Murray, C. J. L., Salomon, J. A., Mathers, C. D., and Lopez, A. D. (2002). *Summary Measures of Population Health: Concepts, Ethics, Measurement and Applications*. Geneva: World Health Organization.

Musgrove, P., Zeramdini, R., and Carrinb, G. (2001). *A Summary Description of Health Care Financing in WHO Member Countries. Health, Nutrition and Population (HNP) Discussion Paper*. Available at: http://www1.worldbank.org/hnp/hsd/rm_wg3_paper11.asp (accessed 23/3/06).

National Association of Attorneys General. (1998). *Master Settlement Agreement*. Available at: http://www.naag.org/upload/1032468605_cigmsa.pdf (accessed 23/3/06).

National Institutes of Health (1997). *Genetic Testing for Cystic Fibrosis: NIH Consensus Statement Online 1997* April 14–16, 15(4): 1–37. http://consensus.nih.gov/1997/1997GeneticTestCysticFibrosis106html.htm (Accessed 7/2/06)

National Institutes of Health (2000). *Enhancing the Oversight of Genetic Tests: Recommendations of the SACGT*. Bethesda, MD: Secretary's Advisory Committee on Genetic Testing, NIH.

New, B. (1997). 'The Rationing Debate: Defining a Package of Healthcare Services the NHS is Responsible for'. *British Medical Journal*, 314(7079): 498–502.

Nijsingh, N. (forthcoming). 'The Expansion of Newborn Screening: In Whose Interest?'

Nord, E. (1993). 'The Trade-off Between Severity of Illness and Treatment Effect in Cost-value Analysis of Health Care, *Health Policy*, 24: 227−38.

Nord, E., Richardson, J., Street, A., Kuhse, H., and Singer, P. (1995). 'Who Cares About Cost? Does Economic Analysis Impose or Reflect Social Values?'. *Health Policy*, 34: 79−94.

Nord, E., Pinto, J.L., Richardson, J., Menzel, P., and Ubel, P. (1999). 'Incorporating Societal Concerns for Fairness in Numerical Valuations of Health Programmes'. *Health Economics*, 8: 25−39.

Nozick, R. (1974). *Anarchy, State & Utopia*. New York: Basic Books.

Nuffield Council on Bioethics (1993). *Genetic Screening: Ethical Issues*. London: The Nuffield Foundation.

Nussbaum, M. (1995). *Poetic Justice*. Boston: Beacon Press.

O'Neill, O. (2002). *Autonomy and Trust in Bioethics*. Cambridge: Cambridge University Press.

O'Neill, M. S., Jerrett, M., Kawachi, I. et al. (2003). 'Health, Wealth, and Air Pollution: Advancing Theory and Methods'. *Environmental Health Perspectives*, 111: 1861−70.

Owen, J. W. (2002). 'Globalisation and Public Health'. *World Hospital and Health Service*, 38(1): 1.

Pangle, T. L. (1988). *The Spirit of Modern Republicanism*. Chicago: University of Chicago Press.

Pappas, G., Queen, S., Hadden, W., and Fisher, G. (1993). 'The Increasing Disparity in Mortality between Socioeconomic Groups in the United States, 1960 and 1986'. *New England Journal of Medicine*, 329: 103−9.

Parfit, D. (1991). 'Equality or Priority,' *The Lindley Lecture*. Kansas: Department of Philosophy, University of Kansas.

Parsons, E.P., Clarke, A.J., Hood, K., and Bradley D.M. (2000). 'Feasibility of a Change in Service Delivery: The Case of Optional Newborn Screening for Duchenne Muscular Dystrophy'. *Community Genetics*, 3: 17−23.

Patten, A. (1996). 'The Republican Critique of Liberalism'. *British Journal of Political Science*, 26: 25−44.

Paul, D. (1995). *Controlling Human Heredity: 1865 to the Present*. Atlantic Highlands, NJ: Humanities Press.

Paul, Y. (2004). 'Letter: Herd Immunity and Herd Protection'. *Vaccine*, 22: 301−2.

Paul, Y. and Dawson, A. (2005). 'Some Ethical Issues Arising from Polio Eradication Programmes in India'. *Bioethics*, 19(4): 393−406.

Perdue, W. C., Stone, L. A., and Gostin, L. O. (2003). 'The Built Environment and its Relationship to the Public's Health: the Legal Framework'. *American Journal of Public Health*, 93: 1390−4.

Perdue, W. C., Stone, L. A. and Gostin, L. O. (2004). 'Public Health and the Built Environment: Historical, Empirical and Theoretical Foundations for an Expanded Role'. *Journal of Law Medicine & Ethics*, 31(4): 557.

Pettit, P. (1997). *Republicanism: a Theory of Freedom and Government*. Oxford: Oxford University Press.

Pettit, P. (1998). 'Reworking Sandel's Republicanism'. *Journal of Philosophy*, 95:73—96.

Pocock, J. G. A. (1975). *The Machiavellian Moment: Florentine Political Theory and the Atlantic Republican Tradition*. Princeton, NJ: Princeton University Press.

Pogge, T. (2002). 'Responsibilities for Poverty-Related Ill Health'. *Ethics & International Affairs*, 16(2): 71—9.

Postema, G. J. (1987). 'Collective Evils, Harms and the Law'. *Ethics*, 97(2): 414—40.

Postrel, V. (1999). 'The Pleasantville Solution: the War on "Sprawl" Promises "Livability" but Delivers Repression, Intolerance—and More Traffic'. *Reason*, 30(10): 4.

Press, N. and Clayton, E. W. (2000). 'Genetics and Public Health: Informed Consent Beyond the Clinical Encounter', in M. J. Khoury, W. Burke, and E. J. Thomson (eds.) *Genetics and Public Health in the 21st Century: Using Genetic Information to Improve Health and Prevent Disease*. Oxford: Oxford University Press, pp. 505—26.

Purdy, L. (1999). 'Genetics & Reproductive Risk: Can Having Children be Immoral?', in H. Kuhse and P. Singer (eds.) *Bioethics*. Oxford: Blackwell, pp. 123—9.

Putnam, R. D. (1995). 'Bowling Alone Revisited'. *The Responsive Community*, (Spring), 1822—32.

Putnam, R. D. (2000). *Bowling Alone*. New York: Simeon and Schuster.

Quetel, C. and Braddoch, J. (1992). *The History of Syphilis*. Baltimore, MD: Johns Hopkins University Press.

Ramsay, J., Richardson, J., Carter Y. H., Davidson, L. L., and Feder, G. (2002). 'Should Health Professionals Screen Women for Domestic Violence? Systematic Review'. *British Medical Journal*, 325: 314—18.

Rawls. J. (1971). *A Theory of Justice*. Cambridge, MA: Harvard University Press.

Reynolds, C. (1995). *Public Health Law in Australia*. Sydney: Federation Press.

Reynolds, C. (2003). 'Public Health Law in the New Century'. *Journal of Law and Medicine*, 10: 435—41.

Risse, M. (2005). 'How Does the Global Order Harm the Poor?'. *Philosophy and Public Affairs*, 33: 349—76.

Robbins, C. (1959). *The Eighteenth Century Commonwealth Man*. Cambridge, MA: Harvard University Press.

Robbins, L. (1962). *An Essay on the Nature and Significance of Economic Science*. London: Macmillan.

Roberts, M. J. and Reich, M. R. (2002). 'Ethical Analysis in Public Health'. *Lancet*, 359(9311): 1055—9.

Roemer, J. (1993). 'A Pragmatic Theory of Responsibility for the Egalitarian Planner'. *Philosophy & Public Affairs*, 22: 146—66.

Rogot, E., Sorile, P. D., Johnson, N.J., and Schmitt, C. (eds.) (1992). *A Mortality Study of 1.3 Million Persons by Demographic, Social, and Economic Factors: 1979—1985 Follow-up.* Bethesda, MD: National Institutes of Health.

Rose, G. (1985). 'Sick Individuals and Sick Populations'. *International Journal of Epidemiology*, 14: 32—8.

Rose, G. (1992). *The Strategy of Preventive Medicine.* Oxford: Oxford University Press.

Ross, L. F. (2002). 'Predictive Genetic Testing for Conditions that Present in Childhood'. *Kennedy Institute of Ethics Journal*, 12(3): 225—44.

Rothstein, M. (2002). 'Rethinking the Nature of Public Health'. *Journal of Law, Medicine & Ethics*, 30: 144—9.

Saah, A. (1996). 'The Epidemiology of HIV and AIDS in Women' in R.R. Faden and N.E. Kass (eds.) *HIV, AIDS, and Childbearing.* New York: Oxford University Press, pp. 9—11.

Salisbury, D. & Begg, N. (eds.) (1996). *Immunisation Against Infectious Diseases.* London: HMSO.

Sandel, M. (1984). *Democracy and its Discontents: America in Search of a Public Philosophy.* Cambridge, MA: Harvard University Press.

Savulescu, J. (1995). 'Rational Non-interventional Paternalism: Why Doctors Ought to Make Judgments on What is Best for their Patients'. *Journal of Medical Ethics*, 21: 327—31.

Scally, G. (2002). 'Too Much Too Young? Teenage Pregnancy is a Public Health, not a Clinical, Problem'. *International Journal of Epidemiology*, 31:554—5.

Scanlon, T. (1998). *What We Owe to Each Other.* Cambridge, MA: The Belknap Press/Harvard University Press.

Scheper-Hughes, N. (1993). 'AIDS, Public Health, and Human Rights in Cuba'. *Lancet*, 342: 965—7.

Schön, D. A. (1983). *The Reflective Practitioner.* New York: Basic Books.

Selgelid, M., Battin, M., and Smith, C. B. (eds.) (2006). *Ethics and Infectious Disease.* Oxford: Blackwell.

Shal, D. J. (ed.) (1996). *Cystic Fibrosis.* London: BMJ Publishing Group.

Shattuck, L. (1850). *Report of the Massachusetts Sanitary Commission.* Cambridge, MA: Harvard University Press.

Shickle, D. (1999). 'The Wilson and Jungner Principles of Screening and Genetic Testing', in R. Chadwick, D. Shickle, H. Ten Have, and U. Wiesing (eds.) *The Ethics of Genetic Screening.* Dordrecht: Kluwer, pp. 1—34.

Singer, P. (1972). 'Famine, Affluence and Morality'. *Philosophy and Public Affairs*, 1(3): 229—43.

Singer, P. A., Benatar, S. R., Bernstein, M. et al. (2003). 'Ethics and SARS: Lessons from Toronto'. *British Medical Journal*. 327(7427): 1342–4.

Skinner, Q. (1978). *The Foundations of Modern Political Thought*. 2 vols. Cambridge: Cambridge University Press.

Skinner, Q. (1997). *Liberty Before Liberalism*. Cambridge: Cambridge University Press.

Skrabanek, P. (1990). 'Why is Preventive Medicine Exempted from Ethical Constraints?'. *Journal of Medical Ethics*, 16: 187–90.

Solomon, J. and Murray, C. (2002). 'A Conceptual Framework for Understanding Adaptation, Coping, and Adjustment in Health State Valuations,' in C. Murray, J. Solomon, C. Mathers, and A. Lopez, *Summary Measures of Population Health: Concepts, Ethics, Measurement and Applications*. Geneva: WHO.

Solomon, J. and Murray, C. (2002). 'Estimating Health State Valuations Using a Multiple-method Protocol,' in C. Murray, J. Solomon, C. Mathers, and A. Lopez (eds.) *Summary Measures of Population Health: Concepts, Ethics, Measurement and Applications*. Geneva: WHO.

Spurrier, N. J., Sawyer, M.G., Clark, J. J., and Baghurst, P. (2003). 'Socio-economic Differentials in the Health-related Quality of Life of Australian Children: Results of a National Study'. *Australian and New Zealand Journal of Public Health*, 27: 27–33.

Srinivasan, S., Dearry, A., and O'Fallon, L. R. (2003). 'Creating Healthy Communities, Healthy Homes, Healthy People: Initiating a Research Agenda on the Built Environment and Public Health'. *American Journal of Public Health*, 93: 1446–50.

Stoto, M. A., Almario, D. A., and McCormich, M. C. (1999). *Reducing the Odds: Preventing Perinatal Transmission of HIV in the United States*. Washington, DC: National Academy Press.

Sullivan, W. M. (1982). *Reconstructing Public Philosophy*. Berkeley, CA: University of California Press.

Sunstein, C. R. (1993). 'The Enduring Legacy of Republicanism', in. S. E. Elkin and K. E. Soltan (eds.) *A New Constitutionalism: Designing Political Institutions of a Good Society*. Chicago: University of Chicago Press.

Sunstein, C. (2005). *Laws of Fear: Beyond the Precautionary Principle*. Cambridge: Cambridge University Press.

Szreter, S. (1988) 'The Importance of Social Intervention in Britain's Mortality Decline c.1850–1914: A Re-interpretation of the Role of Public Health', *Social History of Medicine I*, 1 April, pp. 1–37.

Taylor, C. (1985). *Philosophical Papers*. 2 vols. Cambridge: Cambridge University Press.

Temkin, L. (1993). *Inequality*. Oxford: Oxford University Press.

Tobey, J. A. (1939). 'Public Health in New York State: Report of the New York State Commisssion'. *Public Health Law*. New York: The Commonwealth Fund, p. 57.

Tobin, J. (2005). 'The Challenges and Ethical Dilemmas of a Military Medical Officer Serving with a Peacekeeping Operation in Regard to the Medical Care of the Local Population'. *Journal of Medical Ethics*, 31: 571−4.

Tramont, E. C. (2004). 'The Impact of Syphilis on Humankind'. *Infectious Disease Clinics of North America*, 18: 101−10.

Tramont, E. C. (2005). 'Treponenion Pallidum (Syphilis)', in G. L. Mandell, J. E. Bennett, and R. Dolin, (eds.) *Principle and Practice of Infectious Diseases*. Philadelphia, PA: Elsevier Churchill Livingstone, p. 2781.

Tsuchiya, A. (2000) 'QALYS and Ageism: Philosophical Theories and Age Weighting'. *Health Economics*, 9: 57—68.

Turnbull, C. M. (1972). *The Mountain People*. New York: Simon and Schuster.

Ulmer, J.B. and Liu, M.A. (2002). 'Ethical Issues for Vaccines and Immunization'. *Nature Reviews: Immunology*, 2: 291−6.

US Department of Energy (2002). Office of Science Genome Program. 'Genetic Disease Profile: Cystic Fibrosis'. Available at: http://www.ornl.gov/sci/techresources/Human_Genome/posters/chromosome/cf.shtml (accessed 7/2/06).

US National Library of Medicine/National Institute of Health (2004). Medline Plus, Medical Encyclopedia, Congenital Syphilis. Available at: www.nlm.nih.gov/medlineplus/ency/article/001344.htm (accessed 18/2/06).

US Public Health Service (1999). *The Surgeon General's Call To Action To Prevent Suicide*. Washington, DC: Department of Health and Human Services.

Van den Hoven, M.A. (2006) *Reasonable Morality: Commonsense Concepts of Reasonableness in the Debate on the Limits of Morality*. Utrecht: Zeno.

Van den Hoven, M. and Verweij, M. F. (2003). 'Should we Promote Influenza Vaccination of Health Care Workers in Nursing Homes? Some Ethical Arguments in Favor of Immunization'. *Age & Ageing*, 32: 487−9.

Van Gelderen, M. and Skinner, Q. (eds.) (2002). *Republicanism: a Shared European Heritage*. 2 vols. Cambridge: Cambridge University Press.

Verweij, M. F. (1999). 'Medicalization as a Moral Problem for Preventive Medicine'. *Bioethics*, 13: 89−113.

Verweij, M. F. (2000). *Preventive Medicine Between Obligation and Aspiration*. Dordrecht: Kluwer.

Verweij, M. F. (2005). 'Obligatory Precautions against Infection'. *Bioethics*, 19(4): 323−35.

Verweij, M. F. and van den Hoven, M. A. (2005). 'Influenza Vaccination in Dutch Nursing Homes: Is Tacit Consent Morally Justified?'. *Medicine, Health Care and Philosophy*, 8: 89−95.

Wakefield, A. J., Murch, S. H., Anthony, A. et al. (1998). 'Ileal-lymphoid-nodular hyperplasia, Non-specific Colitis, and Pervasive Developmental Disorder in Children'. *Lancet*, 351: 637−41.

Walker, D. G. and Walker, G. J. A. (2002). 'Forgotten but not Gone: The Continuing Scourge of Congenital Syphilis'. *Lancet Infectious Disease*, 2: 432−6.

Walsh, V. (1996). *Rationality, Allocation, and Reproduction*. Oxford: Clarendon Press.

Walzer, M. (1983). *Spheres of Justice: a Defense of Pluralism and Equality*. London: Basic Books.

Walzer, M. (1987). *Interpretation and Social Criticism*. Cambridge, MA: Harvard University Press.

Warner, K. E. (2000). 'The Economics of Tobacco: Myths and Realities'. *Tobacco Control*, 9; 78−89.

Wasserman, D., Bickenbach, J., and Wachbroit, R. (eds.). (2005). *Quality of Life and Human Difference*. Cambridge: Cambridge University Press.

Weiler, P. C., Hiatt, H., Newhouse, J. P. et al. (2000). *A Measure of Malpractice Medical Injury, Malpractice Litigation, and Patient Compensation*. Cambridge, MA: Harvard University Press.

Wikler, D. (1978). 'Persuasion and Coercion for Health: Ethical Issues in Governmental Efforts to Change Life-styles'. *Milbank Memorial Fund Quarterly*, 56(3): 303−38.

Wikler, D. (1987). 'Personal Responsibility for Illness', in T. Regan and D. Van DeVeer (eds.) *Health Care Ethics*. Philadelphia: Temple University Press.

Wikler, D. (1999). 'Can we Learn from Eugenics?' *Journal of Medical Ethics*, 25(2): 183−94.

Wikler, D. (2004). 'Personal and Social Responsibility for Health', in S. Anand, F. Peter, and A. Sen (eds.) *Public Health, Ethics, and Equity*. Oxford: Oxford University Press, pp. 109−34.

Wilfond, B. S. and Thomson, E. J. (2000). 'Models of Public Health Genetic Policy Development' in M. J. Khoury, W. Burke, and E. J. Thomson (eds.), *Genetics and Public Health in the 21ˢᵗ Century*. New York: Oxford University Press.

Wilkinson, R. G. (1996). *Unhealthy Societies: the Afflictions of Inequality*. London: Routledge.

Wilkinson, S. (1999). 'Smokers' Rights to Health Care: Why the Restoration Argument is a Moralising Wolf in a Liberal Sheep's Clothing'. *Journal of Applied Philosophy*, 16: 255−69.

Williams, A. (1997). 'Intergenerational Equity: an Exploration of the 'Fair Innings' Argument'. *Health Economics*, 6: 117−32.

Williams, B. (1973). 'A Critique of Utilitarianism', in J. J. C. Smart and B. Williams. *Utilitarianism For and Against*. Cambridge: Cambridge University Press.

Williams, B. (1981). 'Persons, Character and Morality', in B. Williams (ed.) *Moral Luck: Philosophical Paper 1973−1980*. Cambridge: Cambridge University Press.

Williamson, J. (1997). 'The Washington Consensus Revisited', in L. Emmerij (ed.) *Economic and Social Development into the XXI Century*. Washington, DC: Inter-American Development Bank.

Wilson, J. M. G. and Jungner, G. (1968). *Principles and Practice of Screening for Disease*. Geneva: World Health Organization.

Winslow, C. E. A. (1920). 'The Untilled Fields of Public Health'. *Science*, 51: 23.

Wolff, J. (forthcoming). 'Risk, Fear, Blame, Shame and the Regulation of Public Safety'. *Economics and Philosophy*.

Wolin, S. S. (1968). 'Political Theory: Trends and Goals', in D. S. Sills (ed.) *International Encyclopedia of the Social Science*, vol. 12: 318–31. New York: Macmillan Co.

Wong, M. D., Shapiro, M. F., Boscardin, W. J., and Ettner, S. L. (2002). 'Contribution of Major Diseases to Disparities in Mortality'. *New England Journal of Medicine*, 347: 1585–92.

Wood, G. S. (1972). *The Creation of the American Republic, 1776–1787*. New York: Norton.

WHO (World Health Organization) (1946). Constitution of the World Health Organization, New York, 22 July. Available at: http://www.who.int/governance/en/ (accessed: 28/1/06).

WHO (World Health Organization) (1983). International Health Regulations. Available at: http://www.who.int/csr/ihr/current/en/(accessed 23/3/06).

WHO (World Health Organization) (2000a). *Obesity: Preventing and Managing the Global Epidemic*. Geneva: WHO.

WHO (World Health Organization) (2000b). World Health Report 2000. Geneva: WHO.

WHO (World Health Organization) (2002a). *Current and Future Long-Term Care Needs*. Geneva: WHO.

WHO (World Health Organization) (2002b). *Lessons for Long-Term Care Policy*. Geneva: WHO.

WHO (World Health Organization) (2002c). *State of the World's Vaccines and Immunization*. Geneva: WHO.

WHO (World Health Organization) (2003). *Ethical Issues in Long-Term and Home-Based Care*. Geneva: WHO.

WHO (World Health Organization) (2004). *The Millennium Development Goals and Tobacco Control*. Geneva: WHO.

WHO (World Health Organization) (2005). *HIV/AIDS Epidemiological Surveillance Report for the WHO African Region: 2005 Update*. Geneva: WHO.

INDEX

age
and justice 82–83, 88, 117–118
as risk factor 135–135
aggregation 5, 11, 22–24, 35–36, 47–51, 56, 64, 111–128, 141, 182, 187–190
autism 95–96, 110

beneficence/non-maleficence 166–168
Bentham, J. 24, 35, 41

CEA (cost-effectiveness analysis) 82–83, 111–128
choice 18, 34–35, 62, 65, 95–110, 131–133, 145, 153–5, 157–158, 172, 180–183, 190, 193, 204–214
coercion 2, 34, 103, 105, 158
collective action 21, 25–27, 50, 137, 191
collective goods and ideals 136–137; see also public goods
collective intervention 21, 25–27
common good 27–28, 32–34, 46–47, 50, 52, 58, 61–64
as different from aggregated interests 36, 47
in relation to civic virtue 46–47
communitarianism 8, 38, 43
consequentialism 6, 8, 119, 143
contact tracing 150
contractarianism 8, 31, 35, 42, 52, 56, 183,
contractualism 120, 142–143
convergent and congruent interests 136–137
cystic fibrosis (CF) 146, 149–158, 105

democracy 33, 36, 39, 52, 64, 71, 95–97, 106, 109, 182–183, 195
determinants of health 15–18, 20, 23–24, 74, 78, 90–91, 134, 138–139, 191–196
Duchenne Muscular Dystrophy 200–201, 215–217, 223

egalitarianism 120–121
epidemic 5, 51, 76, 88, 137
equity 83, 112–114, 124–128
social economic inequities 70, 72–74, 77,89–90
environmental health inequities 86
global health inequities 89–91
eugenics 87
externalities 50, 190

Feinberg, J. 34, 166–167, 183
free riders 11, 50, 55, 99, 161, 166, 173–177

Gonorrhea 146
government responsibilities/obligations 11, 15, 18–21, 25, 27, 33, 39, 42, 54, 62–77, 80, 90, 101, 117, 154–155, 180–3, 186, 195, 204

harm to others (harm principle) 6, 11, 27, 34, 70–72, 99, 133, 136, 161, 166–177, 180, 183–187, 190–191, 194
health education; see health promotion
health factors; see determinants of health
health information; see health promotion
health measurement 83–84
health promotion 3, 7, 26–27, 37, 57, 61, 69–71, 77, 80, 100, 181–182, 187, 194
health; see also public health
WHO definition of health 17
hepatitis B 22, 28–29, 146
herd protection 5, 11, 26, 51, 65, 135–136, 160–178
distinguished from herd immunity 162–163
HIV/AIDS 4, 7, 57, 76, 82, 87–89, 92, 146–147, 157–9
human rights 31, 67, 81
Huntington's disease 146

influenza (flu) 4, 10, 129–144
    avian flu 87, 133, 140
informed consent 102, 151, 153, 157,
    197–212

Kant, I. 174–5

liberalism 6, 8, 31–42, 47, 53–58, 59, 61, 167,
    177, 182–184, 195
libertarianism 31, 61–62, 74

Machiavelli 38, 40
measles 95–96, 99; see also MMR
Mill, J.S. 167–167, 183
MMR (Measles-Mumps-Rubella)
    vaccine 95–101, 106–110
mumps 95–96, 99; see also MMR

nursing homes 135–139

pandemic 4, 87, 92
paternalism 34, 154, 156–157, 167, 180, 183
phenylketonuria (PKU) 146, 200, 207
pluralism 43–44, 182–183, 195
population health 66–8, 78–94
precautionary principle 49, 108–109
preferences 83–84, 114, 179–197, 211
public (the) 24, 36, 48, 51, 53–56
public good(s) 4–6, 24–27, 50–51, 64, 68,
    95, 106, 160–178, 190–196
    vs private goods 5, 24–27
    defined 24–25, 50, 164–165
public health
    definition 9, 13–29
    legal tools to protect public
        health 68–78
    values of public health 66–67
    as distinct from clinical medicine 2–3,
        35, 79–81, 146, 198, 210
    public health ethics 1–12, 27–29; 30–58
    public health
        interventions/practice 2–5, 9, 11,
        13–29, 68–78, 193–194
    public health law 59–77
    public health problem 4, 13–8, 30, 35,
        69, 194
    public health professionals 2, 34–5, 37,
        57, 66
    public health programmes 3, 5, 10, 130,
        143–144, 183

quarantine 3–4, 34, 145, 162

Rawls, J. 34, 121, 164, 175
republicanism 30–58
responsibility 19, 29, 32, 34, 50, 54, 62–6,
    79–81, 97, 99–103, 137, 185, 187, 197,
    212
    individual responsibility 62, 80–81
    collective responsibility 19, 62, 197
    professional responsibility 141
Rose, G. 21, 61, 91, 129
rubella 95–96, 99, 146, 164; see also MMR

SARS (Severe Acute Respiratory
    Syndrome) 3–4, 87, 140, 145
Scanlon, T. 120, 142
scientific realism 95–110
screening 7–8, 16, 25–26, 87, 123, 129–130,
    149–158, 197–212
    newborn/neonatal 149, 197–212
    carrier screening 152
    cancer screening 8, 26, 130
sickle cell anemia 146
smoking 7, 11, 14, 26, 70–71, 74, 80, 117,
    179–197
    passive smoking 181, 183, 185–187
syphilis 146, 148–159
    testing of 150–153
    screening for 150

taxes 26, 62, 69–70, 77, 174, 181–182
Tay-Sachs 146
testing 29, 76, 87, 148–159, 200–201
    genetic testing 152, 154, 200
    premarital testing 148
Tragedy of Commons 51–3, 65
travelling 87, 100, 170, 173

utilitarianism 31, 35, 38, 41, 43, 47, 119–120,
    132, 140, 182, 189, 196

vaccination (immunisation) 3, 5–7, 10–11,
    22, 25–6, 28–29, 51, 61, 65, 92, 96–110,
    115, 129–145, 160–177
vaccine 3–4, 10, 25, 75, 96–103, 106–107,
    110–3, 119, 133, 159–165, 168–171, 174
virtues 32, 44–46, 48
    civic virtue 32, 40–47, 52–58

Wilson and Jungner 155, 200, 211